RECLAIM YOUR LIFE

IN SEVEN SIMPLE STEPS

The advice in this book may not be suitable for everyone. Always consult your doctor before changing your diet or lifestyle.

This book contains a small number of affiliate links. If you buy through a link, the author will receive a small commission, but you will not pay any more. All products are genuine recommendations used by the author and/or her clients.

Since this is science, we reserve the right to alter or edit our stance as new data comes out. As with science, new data often comes out and facts can be proven differently. For now, however, these are facts we are confident about based on our research as well as our work that we do with our clients.

This book is dedicated to the memory of my late father, whose long battle with depression taught me the importance of positivity, giving and health.

I have written this to show as many people as possible that you can take back control of your life in terms of happiness, lifestyle, nutrition and movement. It can be simple and enjoyable and reap genuinely life-changing results.

It will have been worthwhile if just one person finds health and happiness through my words.

Pippa Hill

*"Don't ask yourself what the world needs.
Ask yourself what makes you come alive, and
go do that, because what the world needs is
people who have come alive."*
- Howard Thurman

Client Testimonials (all available online):

"The decision to work with Pippa is one of the best ones I've made with my health and fitness. During my 4 weeks of working with her, I lost half a stone in weight! With her expert knowledge and support, I overhauled my lifestyle (what I eat, when I eat and the best time to exercise). I'll continue with this journey to get to my ideal weight/body shape. I'd highly recommend Pippa if you want to lose weight sustainably and for the long term. Thank you Pippa for everything :)..." - Seun Odusanya

"Pippa's nutritional knowledge is superb. The food is so easy for my busy life. The exercise no gym needed I've lost a stone of menopausal weight gain in a couple of months. Now on the way to getting back to my low weight from 30's. Feeling happy and healthy. Highly recommended..." - Julia O'Gorman

"Quite simply the best way I have ever tried to lose weight! Pippa is brilliant explaining the science behind food and eating. Weekly chats and continuous encouragement really help along with new Information to reach that goal. After 8 weeks I have lost 1 stone, and feel guilty if I don't do my morning exercises. Thats a new me! For me, this has been a lifestyle change not a diet. I can feel the change in my body shape and my husband and friends started commenting after only a few weeks. I cant thank Pippa enough for showing me the way to a healthy, happier me...." - Angela Croxford

"Pippa has been truly amazing at guiding me through the best and healthiest ways to lose weight. I had tried diets in the past, healthy eating etc but nothing

seemed to work. I contacted Pippa and joined her for an 8 week programme - with her expert knowledge and support, I overhauled my lifestyle (what I eat, when I eat and the best time to exercise) and I'm delighted that I have lost 3 stone! I couldn't of done it without her and I couldn't recommend The Weight Loss Guru more highly!" - Hayley Crowe

"Pippa is effective, supportive and persistent. I'm down three stone (in 6 months) thanks to her sensible and facts-based method. I really wanted to lose weight, and I also knew I needed expert help - Pippa provided that in the form of weekly check-ins, routines, recipes, exercises and advice. She's great!" - Sarah Finke

"Pippa was great at providing all the information you need to make better choices in diet and lifestyle. Her coaching sessions were useful and kept me on track to reach my goals. I lost 10kg in just over 3 months even with long haul business travel which was amazing. Easy to understand and worked around a busy schedule, family and work commitments. I even kept it up on holiday." - Nichole Gandemer

"When you search for answers for 3 years, failing, starting again and failing again and then this incredible lady comes along and gets it all fixed in 3 weeks - that feels magical. Pippa is a real deal in all things fitness, healthy lifestyle and of course weight loss. 5kg off and feeling fantastic- and only regret is to why I didn't meet Pippa earlier in my life to kick start this life style earlier and feel happy healthy and energetic." - Marina Lyons

"It's not an exaggeration to say that Pippa has changed my life. I've struggled with my weight, and with emotional eating as long as I can remember. I'd got to a point where I despaired. I had tried every diet going. And I usually lasted about four weeks before falling spectacularly off the wagon and piling all the weight back on. And then a friend who was the same age as me had a heart attack. Something had to change. Pippa has changed not just what I eat, but when I eat, and how I exercise. I'm always interested in the evidence, and everything that Pippa does is backed up by science. I am 23lbs down and the same weight I was when I got married. 18 years ago. I ran my fastest 5k in 20 years last week. And I'm stronger, and fitter than I've ever been. She's a marvel and she's given me a system I can use for the rest of my life." - Lisa Quinn

"I cannot recommend highly enough. When I found Pippa I thought if I don't do something I am only going to continue to gain weight. Lockdown, menopause and depression sent me into a downward spiral and none of my attempts to get back on track worked anymore. Pippa gave me the tools and. motivation to do what I needed to do and I feel back to my old self again after only 2 months. Thank you! X" - Debbie Hryb

"I was quite sceptical when I signed up to the 6 week program with Pippa - after all, I tried so many diets and I thought I was quite clued up about nutrition. The program, Pippa's insights and her help have been the best gift I've ever done to myself. For the first time ever I've been able to feel ok about my body and that was through a lifestyle change that is easy to carry on after the program, rather than a quick fix diet. Super recommended!" - Cecilia Manduca

"I lost 23 lbs with Pippa and have a whole new way to live! All my lockdown weight is gone. It's easy to follow and based on science. Thanks Pippa!" - Korina Holmes

"I met Pippa at a time when I really wanted to lose weight and I almost 'knew' too much to know where to start. She explained very clearly the science behind her approach, busted some myths, and made it very accessible, with great accountability. The weight loss has been rapid, but healthy, and sustainable. I am never going back to where I was." - Selina Lamy

"The weight loss guru Pippa is absolutely amazing and over the past 3 months I have lost 2stone 11lbs by following her plan. I have changed when and what I eat with Pippa's weekly advice and support. Pippa also gives exercises to do to enhance the food pl" - Yvonne Coggins

"What a fabulous, caring and inspirational woman! Pippa is fantastic and a complete life saver. Her knowledge on all things nutrition and being healthy is second to none. She guides you through making realistic lifestyle changes with no faddy diets or tricks. If you want to get healthy and manage your weight, look no further." - Stevie Wicks

"Pippa is a genius! I have lost 3 stone and got my original body back. I love the way Pippa looks at everything.It's a life style change not a diet with not just a focus on what you eat, but when you eat, how to exercise and the mental side of things too! Life changing and worth every penny if you are struggling and unhappy with you weight!" - Nicky Patrick

"I have been working with Pippa for 3 months now and as a result have lost almost 14kg. Her strict no nonsense philosophy was exactly what I was looking for as with the right mental attitude it is easy to work into your daily routine. Pippa was flexible with the package I took and now I really enjoy our monthly check-ins to make sure I am staying in track. A real game changer." - Andy Devey

"A few weeks in and the results are amazing! 16KG down already. Pippa's no nonsense approach really works and knowing that you you will see her every week keeps you on track :)" - Savva Zacharia

"Cheesy as it sounds, Pippa has changed my life. I've lost 40lb in 4 months, all while socialising and enjoying food. After years of food guilt and dieting, a *fortune on PTs and fads, for the first time in my life I feel in control. Pippa had taught me so much about nutrition and my body that the right choices come easy now with no calorie counting or obsessing."* - The Fooks

You can access **Additional Resources** such as my delicious recipes, easy workout videos, and links to products (which you can also find spread throughout the book), and much more besides, by scanning this QR code:

Your password is TWLGBOOKRYL

You'll only need to leave a first name and an email address so we can send you everything, and we never share your details with any third parties.

Contents

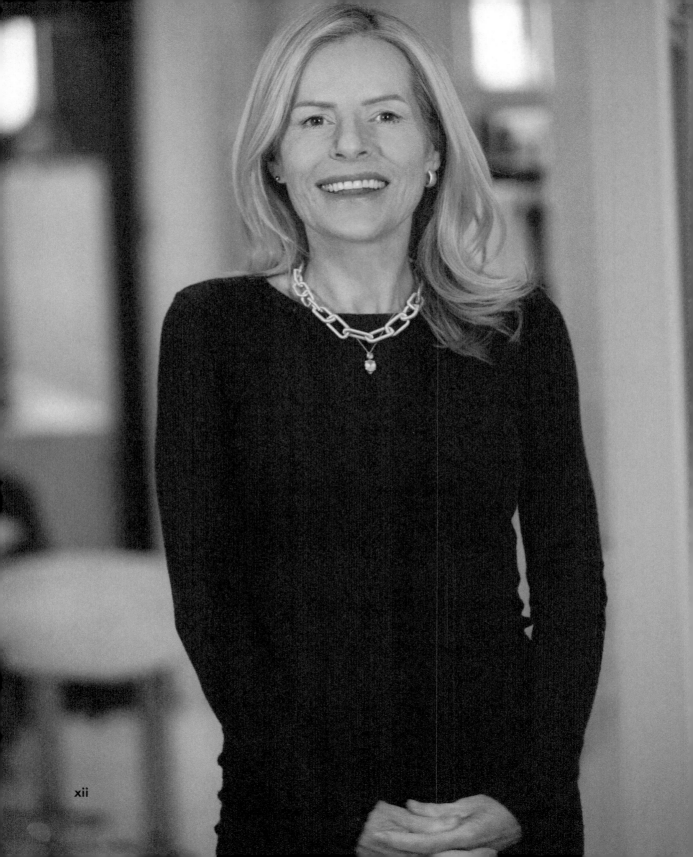

Introducing the RECLAIM Your Life Program

"If you feel heavy in the body you can feel heavy in the head, the heart and the soul. If you feel light you can fly."
Pippa Hill

Congratulations! By opening this book, you have taken the first small step on your journey to a healthier, happier, slimmer life - forever. All you need to do is commit to keeping walking down that path. If you stick to the plan, you will see excellent results within just a few months, and those results will last for the rest of your life.

How can I possibly make that promise? Quite simply, I've had a lot of practice! They say it takes 10,000 hours to become an expert in something. Well, in the last 12 years, I have spent over 43,000 hours helping clients to lose weight. I have worked one-to-one with over 2000 people alone in the last two years. That has given me considerable experience, allowing me to develop methods that are tried, tested and based on evidence and results. Most of my work has been coaching people one-to-one, which means I have seen how my advice plays out in the real world. I know that different people have different challenges, and I have helped them overcome them regardless of their situation. I don't offer a prescriptive diet. Instead, I develop a bespoke plan tailor-made for everyone, incorporating fitness, psychology, and nutrition. If you want some inspiration, look at the testimonials on my website. You will find lots of real-life people who have undergone incredible transformations. In this book, I will show you how to craft your weight loss journey - and I promise it will be easier than you think!

My method is the easiest way to get the body shape you want. It is not a diet. There are no weird rules, no fads, no cutting out food groups, no tracking, and no measuring or counting. You don't even have to set foot in a gym unless you want to. Instead, you will learn more about how your body works and understand why some foods help you become leaner and others don't. You will know why eating at certain times can be helpful and how to achieve that in your busy life. You will even understand that sometimes you can go completely off-plan and how to rein it back in again afterwards. That knowledge puts you back in control of your body and gives your life back. I have around 1000 clients a year who lose 1st (over 6kg) per month and reclaim their lives - you could do the same.

Why do you want to lose weight? You may want to drop 5kg and look stunning for a special occasion, or you've been told that you have pre-diabetes and weight loss helps. It could be that you want to reduce the risk of developing certain cancers or look forward to playing football with your grandchildren many years from now. Whatever your reason, maintaining a healthy weight is a vital part of being happy in life.

I learnt the importance of positivity early in life. My father struggled with manic depression and sadly died through suicide. Of course, mental illness can affect anyone, but the experience taught me that happiness must come from within. Other close relatives have bipolar disorder and psychosis. This program addresses positivity and finding your purpose. I incorporate well-established cognitive behavioural therapy and neuro-linguistic programming techniques. I have dedicated my life to helping people find happiness, reclaim their lives, and live their best lives.

Remember, Serotonin, which comes from the gut, is a neurotransmitter that stimulates satisfaction, happiness and optimism. Our natural endorphins are produced through standing, moving and exercise. So a healthy lifestyle naturally induces positivity.

Later, when my mother died of cancer, I learnt the astonishing truth about how significantly nutrition affects our health. Healthy eating can reverse 90% of some cancers, cure 90% of most heart conditions and reduce or reverse bloating, intolerances, Alzheimer's, arthritis, type 2 diabetes, dementia, IBS, PCOS, NAFLD, SIBO, SIFO, depression, anxiety, sleep apnoea, acid reflux, headaches, gut inflammation, most skin problems including acne and eczema, blood pressure, cholesterol, hormone issues and weight problems. Obesity is categorically linked to practically every serious health issue there is.

"Good nutrition can reverse cancers (particularly breast and prostate), heart disease, osteoporosis, Alzheimer's, kidney stones and blindness."
T Colin Campbell

Sugar addiction is one of the biggest killers in the world right now. Obesity and type 2 diabetes are prolific. As I write this, 75% of the Western Hemisphere's population is classified as obese or overweight, increasing yearly. In the GCC, this figure could be as high as 80%. In Africa and Asia now, these figures are significantly increasing every year. The forecast is that by 2030, 50% of the UK and US population will be obese. That means that by 2030 half the population in many parts of the world could be suffering from significant health issues and potentially be economically inactive. This crisis is more urgent than even global warming! Perhaps even more worrying for the future is that we have seen a 70% increase in diabetes type 2 in 30 year olds and one in four children now leave primary school obese.

However, the good news is that none of this need to be a problem! All of this can be reversed with a healthy lifestyle, and my program can have you living a better quality of life within weeks.

We have access to so much advice these days. Almost a head explosion of knowledge regarding nutrition, diets, fads and tricks is available to us. Noom, Keto, Slimming World, Weight Watchers, Dukan, calorie counting apps, Cambridge Diet and a million more. The statistics make it clear that these approaches are not working. The internet gives us near-instant access to any of them. Still, the global population is heading quickly towards a significant health crisis. How many times do I have to say diets don't work? By definition, with a diet, you are simply doing something weird or restrictive for a finite amount of time. This is unsustainable, and as soon as you return to normal, all the weight will go back on again, and maybe more.

RECLAIM your life is different. It is not a diet, and it is not prescriptive. I give you food plans, menu plans, and recipes, but they are just for you to use as a reference; to provide you with ideas for delicious food. Food is a pleasure and a privilege. We love food. There are no rules (apart from no telly eating to be discussed later!). I will give you the bigger picture. What foods are best for you to eat and when. All foods are already in your fridge. No supplements, no calorie counting, no weighing, no measuring. Everything is just normal, natural lifestyle eating. No going to the gym.

All my clients say that until they found me, they'd tried everything (diets). Nothing had worked or been sustainable, or they'd done well at the beginning, but then the weight had always gone back on again. The first thing they say every time about this program is how easy it is. I always say – yes, being healthy doesn't need to be hard!? Then they comment how full they feel on my program (I think the many restrictive diets they've tried in the past have given them a fear of hunger). The main comment they make (which makes me cry with happiness) is that it is the first program they've ever done that makes them believe they can maintain it for the rest of their life. That this is working for them, that the fat is falling off, that this is the first thing they can see as a lifestyle they can keep to forever. They comment that this truly is 'life changing'.

We know that the RECLAIM Your Life program can make an enormous difference because it's easy to follow and gives outstanding results. Still, of course, I can only work with a limited number of clients one-to-one. Yet I'm on a mission to help the whole world find happiness, positivity, motivation, fat loss whilst reversing type 2 diabetes and obesity!

That is why I've written this book - to help as many people as possible to reclaim their life, health and happiness. Let's get started!

"If you want to turn a vision into reality, you must give 100% and never stop believing in your dream."
Arnold Schwarzenegger

What makes the RECLAIM program different?

If you are like most of my clients, this isn't the first time you have tried to lose weight. Many people have been on a dieting roller coaster, sometimes for many years. Often it starts with meal plans in magazines, promising a beach body in two weeks. They might lose some weight, but when the two weeks are over, those kilograms soon come back and bring a few more with them.

People then move on to try plans that claim they "are not a diet", even though they come with pages, often whole books, listing foods that are or are not allowed. Everything must be measured and counted, which is only sustainable in the short term. Then there are the meal replacement bars, shakes and ready meals, or the fad diets that cut out whole food groups.

None of these teaches you about healthy nutrition, and eventually, you return to eating "normally". But, unfortunately, that's the same "normal" that put on the weight in the first place. You have yet to learn where you went wrong and have yet to address any emotional problems. Before long, you are right back where you started, feeling more than a little disillusioned with the process.

If this is you, maybe you don't honestly believe that you will ever achieve your ideal body shape. Perhaps you beat yourself up about all the times you have "failed" to lose weight or wondered if it could just be genetics. You might question whether healthy body composition and your dream shape are possible. I can guarantee that it is!

I have worked with thousands of clients in all sorts of situations. I have never failed yet, and I don't intend to start with you. Instead, through the pages of this book, I will walk by your side and support you on this journey. Together, we will get there. I promise!

The first step is to get off the diet roller coaster, and the RECLAIM program does exactly that. There is no strict meal plan, no counting and no weird fads. Instead, you will not be following a meal plan imposed by someone else when the realities of life make it impractical, and you return to what you were doing before. Instead, this program is all about education. You will learn which foods will benefit you most and which are less helpful. You will also learn about timing your meals, the role of exercise and how to address the emotional side of overeating. Finally, you will use a smart scale to determine your body composition. Equipped with this knowledge, you will have the tools to lose weight almost effortlessly and transform your entire lifestyle - forever.

The best thing about this way of life is that you will never be restricted. You can still go to that party, enjoy drinks with friends or have an indulgent lunch. The difference is that instead of feeling you have ruined your journey, you will know what to do next. For example, suppose you get invited to 5 parties the week before Christmas and start seeing weight creeping on. In that case, you will rein it in again and watch the excess fat melt away. That is the whole point of this program. It makes achieving and maintaining a healthy weight easy and stress-free. All you need to do is commit to the plan.

What does your weight mean?

Your weight means very little out of context. All it tells us is how heavy you are, but of course, you are a complete human being, and your weight is made up of many things. You have bones and organs, muscles, subcutaneous fat and visceral fat. A bodybuilder with high muscle mass could weigh the same as someone with a lot of subcutaneous fat, but their health and body shape would be very different. You could even be skinny but have a lot of visceral fat (internal fat deposited around your organs), which would be linked with poor health.

What matters is not your weight. It's the amount and type of fat you have that makes a difference. As a result, we will be aiming for fat loss, not necessarily weight loss. You will discover what your body composition is in chapter 2 by using a smart scale. This is your secret weapon for creating the body you want! Once you know what your weight is made up of, you will know what to do about it.

You might be surprised to hear that you and only you created your current shape. Genetics has minimal influence, but other than that, it's all down to you. I don't say this to make you feel guilty or ashamed, if nobody has ever taught you how to eat for health, then it's hardly your fault that you have gained weight! But the fact remains that your current shape is 80% the result of what you eat and drink, 15% influenced by exercise and only 5% genetics.

This is good news! You are in control of your own body. You can change your eating and exercise habits. Even your genetics don't need to be a life sentence, and I'll talk you through that, too, in this book. After years of feeling trapped by your weight, at the mercy of the latest fad diet, you are now back in control - where you should be.

If you create your current shape, you can create any shape you want. What a powerful thought!

Discovering the Future You

Before we go any further, let's try an exercise. I love to do this with my clients because it is compelling. You can come back to this any time if you want an extra boost to your motivation.

Hold your hand up in front of you and imagine your palm is a magic mirror, reflecting you precisely as you are today. Take a long, hard look and be honest with yourself. What do you see? Are you happy with the reflection? Naturally, you will start with your physical appearance but widen out from there. What about your confidence? Happiness? Health? Do you like the way you appear to the world and your contribution to it? What is your purpose in life?

Since you have bought this book, it's safe to assume that the reflection you see right now is not perfect. But don't worry. This book will help you achieve your goals. It's important to note the things you are unhappy about now, both as motivation and so that you know what changes you want to work towards.

Today you are standing at a fork in the path. You can carry along the old, familiar road you have been on for years. Or you can use this book as your guide and take a new path. Let's walk down each one and see what we find. First, the familiar way. Look at your magic mirror again as it reflects an image of you two years from now. Whatever issues you have with your weight now will only get worse. Are you happy with the reflection you see and the extra weight you have gained? What effect might that weight gain have on your life? Has your health deteriorated? Have you lost confidence? Are you motivational to those around you? Are you inspirational?

Think about what you have eaten in those two years and see the crisp packets, chocolate wrappers and takeaway cartons piled around you. Are there empty bottles too? How many times have you indulged in overeating? Did you enjoy it?

Now we move a little further down the path five years from now. How much weight have you gained? Is your health starting to suffer? Do you not sit next to people on the bus for fear of taking up too much space? Look for chairs without arms so your hips don't get stuck? Can you buy clothes from your favourite shops? How many empty fast-food wrappers are littered around you after another 5 years of your eating habits? Are you excelling at your job, or is your confidence waning with your appearance and health issues?

Ten years into the future, your weight gain has likely continued, and you might now have significant health issues. How old are you? How old are your children? Perhaps you have grandchildren! Do you inspire them? Can you do the things you want to do with them? How many empty bottles and empty snack packets are lying around you now after 10 years of the way you've been eating?

Take some time to think about what you see in the magic mirror. It can be painful, but it is essential to feel that and recognise it for what it is. Change is inevitable. No neutral option lets you stay as you are without ageing a day. You *will* walk down one of these paths. The only question is which one? You have the opportunity now to commit. You can say, "enough is enough!", make a promise to yourself and set off on a new path. You can transform your life.

Let's explore that second path now, gaze into your magic mirror and picture yourself just three months from today. You have been following the plan and reclaiming your life. You have started eating at the correct times and choosing the right foods. You have healed your relationship with food and started moving in the right way for you. In three months, you could have reduced your weight by 15kg. You can see that your fat levels have significantly decreased. Calories are burning, your metabolism is working well, and your health is starting to recover. Already you can see a huge difference, even in as little as three months!

Your commitment has already brought you a long way, but it can take you further. Six months into the future, you have completely transformed yourself! I have had clients lose as much as 30kg to 40kg in six months, although results vary depending on your starting point. But with the right mindset, almost anything is possible. So if you can transform yourself in six months, what do you see in two years? Five years?

Without a shadow of a doubt, you love your reflection now. Feeling confident - you feel and look amazing! You have more energy; those little aches and pains have vanished, and even severe health conditions have been reversed or avoided.

What else do you see? Weight loss has given you the confidence to find a new partner, or helped with fertility issues, and a brood of children surrounds you! You may have earned a promotion or decided to run your own business, and your work has completely taken off. It's amazing what a bit of confidence can do for a person once you feel happy and free in your skin.

Now is the moment. You stand at the crossroads and hold the map in your hands. Forging a new path is always a little uncomfortable initially. Still, you will agree that the destination is more than worth it. I promise you that whenever you look back, you will feel proud of yourself for making the right decision today. You will feel proud for making that commitment and stepping off the well-worn path towards a far brighter future.

Meet Your Fellow Reclaimers

Before we dive into the program, I would like to introduce you to three 'Reclaimers' who will be on this journey with you*. Through them, you will see how the seven principles in the RECLAIM program translate into real life - and how they overcome any obstacles and setbacks they face along the way.

Yasmin

Yasmin is 24 and works from 9-5 in a marketing agency as a junior account manager in central London. Her co-workers are the best part of her job (besides getting paid). They regularly share lunch and get together for girls' nights, which usually involve cocktails and late-night takeaways.

Yasmin is 5kg over her ideal weight, and she's been trying to reduce the shape of her thighs for ages. She spends hours in the gym each week, even choosing exercises to target her thighs, but nothing seems to help. Not only that, but she's also getting thoroughly bored of the kale smoothies that seem to be the only thing her favourite influencer ever consumes.

When Yasmin tried the magic mirror experience, she saw herself still stuck in her agency, in her same life, and still on that mindless, boring exercise bike! So instead, she has committed to melting away her overdeveloped thighs. She now imagines having the confidence to buy an excellent interview suit and apply for her dream job as a social media manager.

David

David is a 57-year-old paramedic working hectic shifts. Although he needs a certain fitness level to do his job, it's easy for the weight to creep on. Especially when the drive-through gives paramedics free lattes, and you need something to get you through the night shift! The pints down the pub in football season probably don't help much. Or the bacon butties and ready meals - well, it has yet to seem worth cooking since his divorce. More effort just for one person!

David's GP has told him he is pre-diabetic, which has scared him into acting. However, in his line of work, he has seen the consequences of neglecting one's health and doesn't want to end up in the back of his own ambulance. One of his patients joked that David was so out of breath he might need the oxygen mask himself. Of course, he made light of it at the time, but he has never been so embarrassed.

David has committed to improving his health, avoiding type 2 diabetes and living a long and healthy life. He wants to be able to play football in the park with any grandchildren he might have.

Sophie

Sophie is right in the thick with young children at home 24/7. She always imagined that by 42, she would have some handle on life, but most days, she is just exhausted and finding she resorts to comfort food to keep her going. She loves her children passionately, but her days are *exhausting*, with never-ending demands, tantrums and emergencies. She longs for five minutes to herself occasionally.

Sophie has never been petite; she always felt uncomfortable at school, which has continued and developed since. She remembers dieting as young as 13. Her life has been a roller coaster of weight loss and gain. Three times in four years, pregnancy weight gain has only made everything worse, and now her doctor says she's morbidly obese. The GP asked if she had "ever considered losing weight" as if she hadn't already tried everything from the cabbage soup diet to weekly weigh-ins in the village hall!

Sophie feels desperate at this point. Nothing has ever worked for her, so she feels very disheartened. However, she's heard from many that this lifestyle program is easy, isn't a diet and gives permanent results. Best of all, you feel full all day! So, she has committed to giving it her all and seeing what happens. Of course, she wants to be pain-free, to get down on the floor, play with her children, and run after a toddler without feeling winded. But, most of all, she's determined to walk into an "ordinary" high street shop and find her size on the rail.

*Sophie, Yasmin and David are fictional. Still, their situations, problems and the solutions they find are authentic and based on my experience working with thousands of individuals.

The time is now; let's do this!

Are you ready to completely transform your life? To make that ideal reflection possible and see it stay that way forever?

This is the moment to make that commitment officially. To make it even more real, I want you to write it down or make a note on your iPhone. When you write a commitment to yourself or take a pen and sign your name to something, it influences your brain and tells your subconscious that you are serious about this.

I (name) _____

I hereby make a commitment to faithfully follow the RECLAIM program, to create the body I want to live in and reclaim my life.

Signed _____

Date _____

Create a 'Reclaim Your Life' note on your phone or grab a notebook that you can use to record your thoughts as you work through this book. At the end of each chapter, you will find questions and prompts to help you take what you have learnt and apply that knowledge to your life. In some ways, the first page is the most important; you commit to your future self here.

Write this down now:

_____

_____

_____

_____

_____

_____

_____

_____

Please take a moment to read what you have written here and let it sink in.

Then, say it out loud if you can. You will never again be the weight you are today! You are on the verge of something extraordinary, and I'm both proud of you and honoured to walk this path with you. You have chosen a magnificent journey to a stunning future.

We have already delayed too long. It's time to get started.

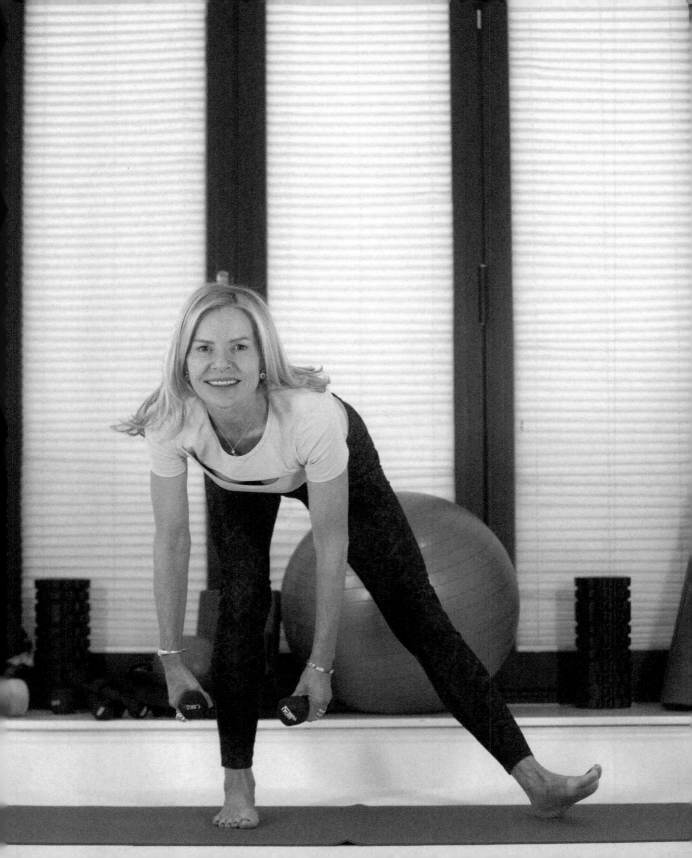

Your Secret Weapon

"If you don't have your health, you don't have anything."
Chuck Pagano

There is a secret weapon in your weight loss journey that's so powerful that everyone should use it. Any nutritionist or dietitian who doesn't tell you about this should not be practising. That secret weapon is a smart scale.

I recommend the RENPHO body fat scale, although there are quite a few on the market. I picked this one because it's affordable and gives you 13 different bits of information. It may be one of the cheapest, but I think it's the best! If you purchase a different model, ensure it gives you all the necessary information. I also love that it connects to a phone app, although some will link to a fitness tracker or smartwatch if you have those.

So, your first step is to order yourself a scale. You can pop over to Amazon, and it will be in your hands tomorrow with next-day delivery. Go on, do it now. I'll wait.

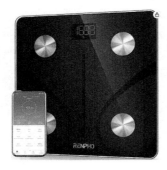 

What is a Smart Scale?

Smart scales are incredibly clever. They use bioelectrical impedance analysis, also referred to as BIA for short, to give you lots of information about your body composition.

This means that the scale sends a small and safe*, electrical charge through your body. It's so tiny that you can't feel it at all. The charge travels at different speeds through different types of body tissue, like fat, bone, water and muscle. This means the scale can measure the way the charge travels and calculate what your body is made of. It's like seeing inside yourself and discovering what is happening, things that even a doctor can't know without the scale.

It is worth noting that smart scales are very safe for the average person. Still, they should be avoided if you have a pacemaker or other medical implant to be on the safe side.

Why is it Important?

Imagine two people weighing the same and being the same height. Standard scales and BMI calculators would say they were the same. But a smart scale reveals hidden secrets.

If someone weighs 80kg, but it's mostly muscle, and they like their muscle levels, then they are happy with that weight. However, if the person standing next to them also weighs 80kg but they have very little muscle and significant fat levels, they might not be so happy with that weight. Some people may have high visceral fat (internal fat wrapped around their organs) and low subcutaneous fat (external fat that you can see on your belly, hips and thighs). Some people might have deficient skeletal muscle and very high muscle mass. You can see how very different they are and how important it might be to track how their body composition changes rather than their total weight. Therefore, the solution to their ideal body shape and size is unique for each person. This program will guide you through what you need to do for your specific issues and needs.

The truth is that a smart scale tells you everything you need to know. My one-to-one clients, and people doing my online course, can send me their readings, and I almost don't need to see them - everything I need to know is there!

We talk about weight loss, but your weight doesn't matter. Let me say that again.

Your Weight Does Not Matter.

What matters is your body composition, not weight loss but fat loss. I often have clients who say they spend ages at the gym, but their weight has increased. However, with a smart scale, you can see that they have increased their muscle mass but lost fat.

Now, I am prepared to be controversial here. Some people like the look of big muscles, and that is great. It's a personal choice. I do have clients, though, who want to look lean. I believe everyone should be free to aim for their ideal body shape. Bulky muscle mass is not always king! If you have bulky muscles and don't like them, I can help you increase your skeletal muscle instead so you healthily have a leaner physique.

One last thing. Don't weigh yourself too often. Once a week is perfect. Your weight can fluctuate by 1 kilo every day. People sometimes want to weigh themselves daily and think it's motivating. You may be one of them. Do you find that not losing weight every day puts you in a bad mood for the whole day? Do you think you might as well eat all those sugary treats since you gained weight anyway? Do you feel that your efforts the day before were wasted?

When you weigh yourself daily, all sorts of things affect the results. Eating late the night before, your hormones, or going to the bathroom can make a big difference. When you weigh yourself daily, those differences can impact your life.

Instead, step on the scales once a week. If you stick to the plan, I can guarantee that you will see the numbers move over a week. You will see the overall picture of becoming healthier every single week. It has always been that way with this program and always will be!

"The best way to predict your health is to create it."
Pippa Hill

Interpreting Your Readout

Your new scales have arrived, and you have downloaded the app and set everything up. When you step on the scales, you will get a whole range of numbers displayed on your phone. The question is, what do they all mean, and what should you do about them?

Weight

This is your total weight; we already know that weight doesn't matter. It is nice to watch the graph track down over the weeks and see the little indicator go from red (obese) through orange (overweight) to green for a healthy weight!

BMI

BMI stands for Body Mass Index. A healthy BMI is from 18.9 to 24.9. A BMI of 25 to 25.9 is overweight. A BMI of 30 or over is obese, and 35 or over is morbidly obese. A BMI of 21 is recommended as the best scientific recommendation.

% Body Fat

This smart scale will tell you what percentage of your body is made up of fat, and you will also get the traffic light colour indicator. From 32% or below, the indicator goes green. The ideal result is approximately 25% for women or 17% for men.

Fat-free Body Weight

This is the weight of all your bones, muscles, blood and organs - everything that isn't fat.

Subcutaneous Fat

Subcutaneous means "under the skin", so this is the fat you can see on your tummy, hips, arms and thighs. It's the kind of fat you want to lose to avoid back issues or hip issues, to fit into that special outfit, and it's also important because it is metabolically inactive. Lean tissue works for you. Every time you move, those chemical reactions occur, and you burn calories, which means a lean person can eat a lot of food without gaining weight. Fat, on the other hand, sits there, metabolically inactive. It doesn't burn calories (levels increase from 30 years old and onwards), so you gain more fat.

High subcutaneous fat is a sign of eating late in the evening, overeating sugar or processed foods or drinking too much alcohol. On the other hand, suppose you start eating right and doing resistance exercises to raise your skeletal muscle. In that case, your subcutaneous fat will go down.

You will find much information on getting your food right in chapter 3. Still, for now, you could have a good size late breakfast, perhaps two hours after you wake up, a large lunch at the usual time and an early dinner at 6pm. Try to make fruit your only snack between meals and aim to cut down on processed grains or sugars such as sweets, bread, rice, pasta and cookies (of course, you can eat these if you're a child, athlete or labourer looking to bulk up). That alone is enough to see the weight start to drop off.

Visceral Fat

This is the most important measurement of all. Visceral fat is internal, wrapped around your organs, which is a significant indicator of health. Visceral fat depends on how much you exercise before breakfast to use your fat reserves; and how much you stand each day. How many monkeys do you see sitting in a chair all day in the wild?! In a very healthy person, this number could be as low as 2, which is a fantastic result. More typically, 6 is good, but anything from 11 down is acceptable. Animals in the wild rarely have visceral fat, just us humans!

If someone is morbidly obese or just obese, this number can be very high such as 20 or even 30. If this is you, I would prioritise lowering it as soon as possible so you can enjoy a longer and healthier life.

Visceral fat is significantly reduced through movement and standing. There is a good deal of information on this in chapter 9.

% Body Water

This is the percentage of your body that is made up of water. Ideally, you want it to be 50% or above. Suppose you want to know more about liquids and the correct carbohydrates that keep you hydrated. In that case, you'll find that information in chapter 7. When we talk about weight loss, we only speak about dry weight. My client's water weight goes up every single week with me. If your water weight is just 40% of you, for example, then 60% of you is dry weight. Imagine if your water level was 60% of you, then only 40% of you is dry weight. That is much easier to lose!

% Skeletal Muscle

Skeletal muscles are the 650 muscles on our body that hold us up, connect our bones and allow us to move. These are the muscles that you control, unlike cardiac muscles (your heart) or the smooth muscles in various organs, which are involuntary. You will notice that in every single person, our subcutaneous fat and skeletal muscle added together always add up to approximately 70% of us. As one goes up, the other always goes down. You will find it much easier to lose weight if you have high skeletal muscle because muscle is a fat burner. However, if you have high subcutaneous fat with low skeletal muscle, you've given yourself a very slow metabolism, and weight gain will continue to increase.

Don't worry; this is all reversible in a very short time. You can eat more and lose weight if you have high skeletal muscle. Do you have friends who can eat everything and still stay lean? Whereas when you look at a bowl of pasta, you feel like you'll put on weight?! The ratio of your subcutaneous fat vs your skeletal muscle explains this. Aim for at least 50% skeletal muscle if you are a man and 40% for a woman. The higher, the better. Lower fat will ultimately lead to better metabolism. You can increase your skeletal muscle by doing resistance exercises: very slow strength exercises involving pushing against something to create that resistance. Resistance exercises you can do any time of day because they target your subcutaneous fat, not visceral, and they burn for 72 hours after you do them, not just whilst you do them. If you think about it, animals in the wild are doing resistance exercises all day long.

Muscle Mass

This is your total muscle weight, including skeletal muscle, cardiac and smooth muscles. Many fitness professionals focus on muscle mass but miss the point. High skeletal muscle means we are just talking about those metabolically active body muscles that can make us look svelte and lean. On the other hand, muscle mass might mean bulky thighs or a heavy heart. This is because when we're very overweight, every time we take a breath, our heart must work that little bit harder for that additional blood flow associated with carrying extra weight. This gives the heart a tiny little scar again and again until the heart does begin to grow, which of course, can lead to health issues in the future.

High muscle mass can be one reason for increased body weight. Some people like high muscle mass, such as large thighs, which is totally up to you. It's simply a personal choice either way.

When you first use your scale, open the home page of the data. You'll find you can click on any of the 13 measurements provided. You will see a low, average, and high indicator line that clarifies where you are and where you should be. This smart scale is impressive! So, if you prefer a leaner body shape, then it's okay to aim to reduce your muscle mass whilst increasing your skeletal muscle.

You can find more information on reducing or balancing your muscle mass in chapter 9.

Bone Mass

Bone mass is not very relevant, but it's nice to see a solid number as it helps avoid osteoporosis. Don't panic if your bone mass drops as you lose weight. That is quite normal. Just as our bone mass will step up to carry the extra weight if we are larger than we want to be, then, in the same way, the bone mass will reduce when we successfully lose that unnecessary weight.

% Protein

This is another important one and something many people need to think about. Protein is crucial for building and repairing all your muscles and organs. Unfortunately, for some people first embarking on their health journey with me, it starts very low. Still, once you start eating healthily and increasing your muscle percentages, you should see this increase weekly.

You particularly want to improve your skeletal muscle if your protein is low. Around 23% of your muscles are protein, so increasing those will help to improve your protein. It would help if you also ate more protein, like fish, meat, peas, Greek yoghurt, protein yoghurt, avocado, hemp seed, chia seeds, pulses, tofu, tempeh & edamame. You want your protein level to be 14% minimum, but nothing wrong with getting it as high as 18%.

BMR

Your BMR is your basal metabolic rate. This is the number of calories you can eat each day to stay the same weight you currently are. You might be surprised by how low this number is, but don't worry, this is a resting rate, and as you become more active, the number goes up. Even standing instead of sitting significantly impacts you, and you'll be surprised by how much you can eat. Standing burns 100 calories per hour!

It also helps to increase your muscle ratio. When you do that, your BMR increases, and you can eat more food without putting on weight.
If you stand for just 5 hours, you can burn 500 calories. You'd have to run 5 miles to achieve the same through exercise. I'd rather stand for 5 hours during an average working day than have to go for a run all the time! Remember, 80% of your body is through the food and drink you consume, only 15% by the exercise you do and 5% through your genetics. It's always your choice, but it's much easier for most to adjust their food and drink rather than aim to burn food off through exercise. This will be our focus. I will also give you significant

exercise advice, but the basis of everything is what you choose to eat and drink.

Remember that you can't exercise off food because of natural muscle wastage once you are over 30 years old. Therefore, you do have to pay significant attention to what you eat and drink.

In the olden days, nutritionists used to say to eat less and exercise more. The classic formula was to take 500 calories off your BMR daily to achieve the necessary 3500 reductions each week to achieve a loss of 1lb of fat per week. But that doesn't allow for the quality of calories rather than quantity, nor for the movement, each person does in a day; hence, that old-fashioned view doesn't hold much sway anymore.

My way on this program is not counting calories, measuring, or weighing. You can eat the most delicious food and plenty of it. More important is the natural timing of your eating and what you eat. It has to be the quality, not the number of calories. But, of course, it does. I can give you ten chocolate biscuits which add up to 1000 calories, or I can give you a portion of chicken and vegetables, a portion of tofu and vegetables and a portion of fish and vegetables, which is also 1000 calories. Please don't tell me those are the same thing. This is why so many diet businesses get it so wrong. Making their clients focus on the quantity, not the quality, can only lead to repetitive failure in weight loss and also an eating disorder. My program reverses eating disorders.

Metabolic Age

Your biometric age is the number of years since you were born. Still, your metabolic age is a much more interesting number. This is the age you have given yourself, which can be 10 years more than your biometric age, depending on how much visceral fat you carry. A very fit and healthy person could be 5 years younger. By taking control of your health and you can reduce your visceral fat; reducing your metabolic age by as much as 10 years! Isn't it worth doing this program just for that alone?!

"In the 20th Century, we have almost doubled life expectancy from forty to seventy, so in the twenty-first century, we should at least be able to double it again to 150."
Yuval Noah Harari

Putting it all together

Seeing all the data laid out like this can be a wake-up call. For others, it's a revelation as they discover things they never knew about themselves. However you are feeling right now, be kind to yourself. Read this chapter over again if you need to. Make sure you understand it and spend some time on your smart scales so you know what each reading means and why.

Everything is connected. As you exercise away your subcutaneous fat, it is replaced by skeletal muscles. When that happens, you will see your protein levels rise. Not only that, but your BMR will also go up - meaning you can eat more without gaining weight. Once you see the numbers move in the right direction, you will never want to let them slide back.

Now that you have this information, you can act. You can change those numbers and see visceral fat going down and protein and water going up. You can see every indicator showing green and a metabolic age that's less than your biometric age. It's going to be fun! Watching all those numbers shift as you gain the perfect body for you and reclaim the life you want to live.

Yasmin, David and Sophie

Yasmin

Yasmin wasn't expecting surprises when she got on her scale for the first time. But she tracks her weight anyway, so she thought she had a good idea of what to expect.

Here are her results:

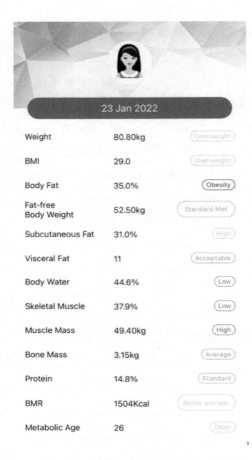

	23 Jan 2022	
Weight	80.80kg	Overweight
BMI	29.0	Overweight
Body Fat	35.0%	Obesity
Fat-free Body Weight	52.50kg	Standard Met
Subcutaneous Fat	31.0%	High
Visceral Fat	11	Acceptable
Body Water	44.6%	Low
Skeletal Muscle	37.9%	Low
Muscle Mass	49.40kg	High
Bone Mass	3.15kg	Average
Protein	14.8%	Standard
BMR	1504Kcal	Below average
Metabolic Age	26	Older

Yasmin knew what her weight would be, and she expected that she would need to lose fat, but she was very surprised by her high muscle mass. Well over half her body weight! With this new knowledge, Yasmin plans to reduce some muscle mass, especially on her thighs, and get the leaner shape she craves. Her visceral fat is acceptable, so her other main goal will be to reduce her subcutaneous fat.

David

After his recent trip to the GP, David was keen to get all the data he could to help him transform his life. So he stepped on the scale, curious and excited to see what he could discover. Mind you, he made sure none of his friends were watching!

Here are his results:

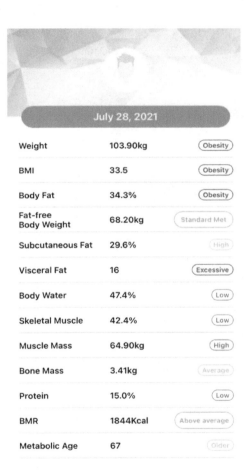

July 28, 2021		
Weight	103.90kg	Obesity
BMI	33.5	Obesity
Body Fat	34.3%	Obesity
Fat-free Body Weight	68.20kg	Standard Met
Subcutaneous Fat	29.6%	High
Visceral Fat	16	Excessive
Body Water	47.4%	Low
Skeletal Muscle	42.4%	Low
Muscle Mass	64.90kg	High
Bone Mass	3.41kg	Average
Protein	15.0%	Low
BMR	1844Kcal	Above average
Metabolic Age	67	Older

Looking at the numbers, David can see many things he can improve. He has bought a water bottle to take to work with him and hopes to see a higher % of water quite quickly. His focus, though, will be reducing visceral and subcutaneous fats. He especially wants to reduce his visceral fat and see his metabolic age decrease - that number was an eye-opener.

Sophie

Sophie was the most nervous of our three reclaimers when she stepped on the scale. The last time she was weighed was by the midwife just before her youngest was born, so she didn't know what to expect.

Here are her results:

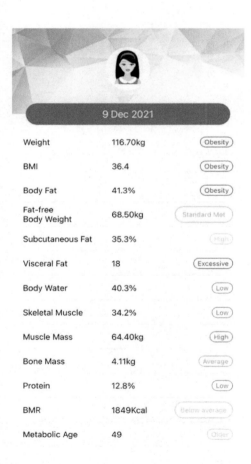

	9 Dec 2021	
Weight	116.70kg	Obesity
BMI	36.4	Obesity
Body Fat	41.3%	Obesity
Fat-free Body Weight	68.50kg	Standard Met
Subcutaneous Fat	35.3%	High
Visceral Fat	18	Excessive
Body Water	40.3%	Low
Skeletal Muscle	34.2%	Low
Muscle Mass	64.40kg	High
Bone Mass	4.11kg	Average
Protein	12.8%	Low
BMR	1849Kcal	Below average
Metabolic Age	49	Older

It turns out that things aren't quite as bad as Sophie feared! She is certainly much heavier than she wants to be, but the gain since her last baby was born is manageable. Sophie's focus will be to reduce both subcutaneous and visceral fats. She plans to walk the children to school and get some cardio in with the buggy simultaneously.

Your Turn

Have you stepped on the scales yet? If not, now is your chance. These scales are excellent. You can set them up to give you weekly or monthly comparisons. You can click on every single piece of data and be informed of where you are versus where you should be. Best of all, you can click on tracking or trends and see a graph of your entire weight history. So once you've been on more than once, every single weigh-in appears on the chart, and you can watch that graph going down and down and down for each measurement that it should. Or up and up for those you want to see an increase in such as proteins, water and skeletal muscle.

Alternatively, grab your notebook, record your starting numbers, and plan your next steps. Keep a space to record your numbers when you hit your goal. Nothing beats seeing those figures side by side! You could copy out a table something like this one:

	Where I started	When I reached my goal
Date:		
Weight:		
BMI:		
Body Fat:		
Fat-free Body Weight:		
Subcutaneous Fat:		
Visceral Fat:		
Body Water:		
Skeletal Muscle:		
Muscle Mass:		
Bone Mass:		
Protein:		
BMR:		
Metabolic Age:		

The thing I will focus on first is:

I will do this by (e.g., exercising three times a week):

My other focus is:

I will do this by:

My first step is (make this simple, it could be reading the next chapter, buying running shoes or planning your meals for tomorrow):

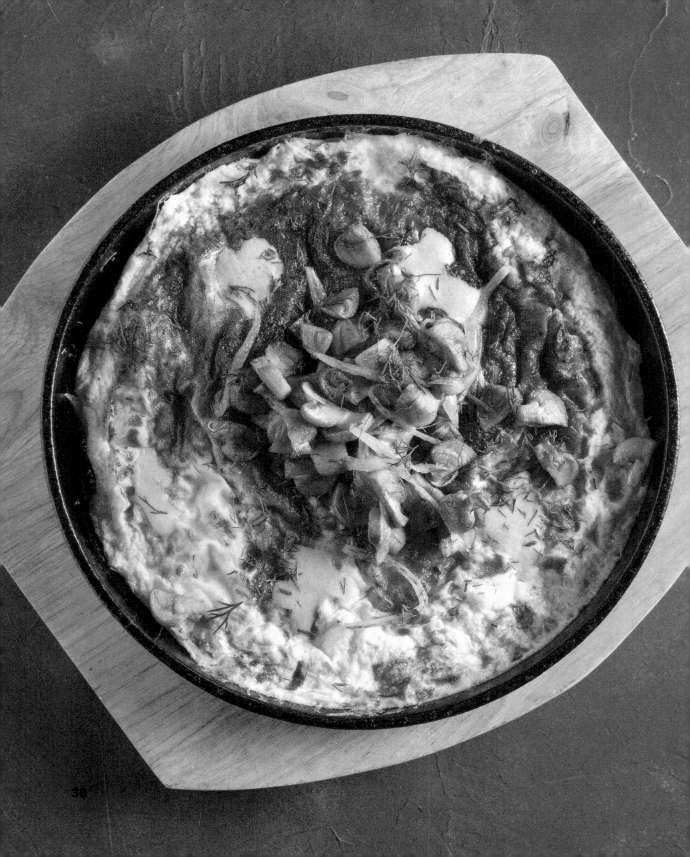

R - Real Food

"Good nutrition: can reverse cancers (particularly breast and prostate), heart disease, strokes, obesity, diabetes, autoimmune disease, osteoporosis, Alzheimer's, kidney stones and blindness."- T Colin Cambell nutritional biochemist

I have promised you seven simple steps to reclaim your life, and this chapter contains step one. By now, I hope you feel motivated and committed to reclaiming your health and the life you want to lead. However, if you have skipped ahead, it is worth taking the time to go back and read chapter 2 when you can. The information there is vital to your success.

RECLAIM is not just the name of this program. It is also an acronym for the seven steps. Of course, we will begin with R, which stands for Real food.

R - Real food

E - Eating time

C - Cut the junk

L - Liquids

A - Alcohol

I - Investigate (emotional eating)

M - Movement

All in a Day's Eating

To start with, let's have a quick look at a typical day's eating. Then when you have an idea of what it looks like, we can talk about the science that makes it work. Remember, this is not about a restrictive meal plan or diet. There are no hard and fast rules, just a framework to help you develop eating habits that support your health and fit your lifestyle.

Breakfast

Focus on proteins for breakfast and aim for a good-sized restaurant portion. You have dozens of delicious possibilities if you are at home and have time to cook. I suggest options such as kippers, avocado, scrambled tofu, scrambled eggs with smoked salmon, mushroom omelette, haddock, harissa beans, mung bean porridge, Greek yoghurt, plant-based yoghurt, chia pots or turkey bacon, and even bacon and eggs. There's so much choice! I would recommend having a maximum of 4 eggs per week because, as they say in *The China Study* and other brilliant scientific health books, eggs are one of the leading causes of health issues in this world. They are cholesterol heavy; a large egg is 180 calories, and they can cause constipation. Wild chickens lay one egg per month, so the fact that we make our chickens lay four eggs per day is insightful!

Of course, many of us are very busy and either eat at work or need more time to cook in the morning. As a single working mother of three and a business owner, I rarely have time to cook breakfast.. If that's you, then I highly recommend my "double yoghurt" bowl. Greek yoghurt (not Greek style, as this is with lactose) is good for you. It has been strained, which means it's lactose-free and is full of natural probiotics and protein to fill you up. FAGE, Waitrose, M&S or Aldi's brand are all excellent options. The only problem is that many people find Greek yoghurt too bitter.

My solution is mixing a pot of Greek yoghurt with a plant-based yoghurt like Alpro or Sojado. The plant-based yoghurts give you extra fibre, more probiotics and the sweet flavour you might need to complement the bitter Greek yoghurt. The combination is gorgeous, and you have a significant portion that will keep you full for hours. If you want to avoid buying individual pots, serve about one-third of a big tub each. It's about 330 grams, but we're not weighing anything. Breakfast needs to be a good size, so you're full up all morning.

Top your yoghurt with a nut and seed blend to increase the health benefits even more. I like to sprinkle on a couple of teaspoons of mixed seeds and nuts like walnuts, almonds, and brazil nuts (good to fight cancer). Then, if you have problems going to the loo, add a teaspoonful of oatmeal. You'll have a hearty breakfast full of healthy fats and proteins. Not only that, but you can also easily throw it together and eat at your desk or wherever you happen to be.

Try and have breakfast roughly two hours after you get up so that you can get some visceral fat burning in before. There are no rules but don't skip breakfast over the age of 40, or your body can start thinking there is a famine and maybe it needs to conserve energy. So even when you're doing shift work, you can work out your timings by allowing that two hours.

We're trying to avoid artificial, processed, starchy foods like toast or cereal, which are full of processed sugars. If you start your morning with processed foods such as these, you will begin the day with an insulin high followed by a crash and hunger cravings. Then, the rest of the day, you will be craving sugars and having peaks and crashes of sugar withdrawals. I will talk more about this later in the chapter.

Lunch

Lunch is the main meal of the day and your opportunity to eat like a king! Here we are going for a generous restaurant-sized portion, plus. Not a restaurant that serves a spoonful of food with a smear of sauce either. I want you to pile your plate high. Think proteins, fats and carbohydrates. This is your energy for the day.

What I mean by this is that you will have your main protein, perhaps salmon, Tofu or chicken, with a big helping of pulses and lots of vegetables. The pulses are brilliant because they fill you up, have lots of fibre, healthy slow-release carbohydrates and are also high in protein - everything you want from food.

When you think of pulses, don't imagine them how they used to be – tasteless tins or dried beans sitting in jars in your grandmother's cupboard. Eating pulses can be daunting for some, but don't panic! You don't have to spend hours boiling chickpeas unless you want to. I certainly don't. As you'll read later in the chapter, pulses are now the trendiest food – the new superfood

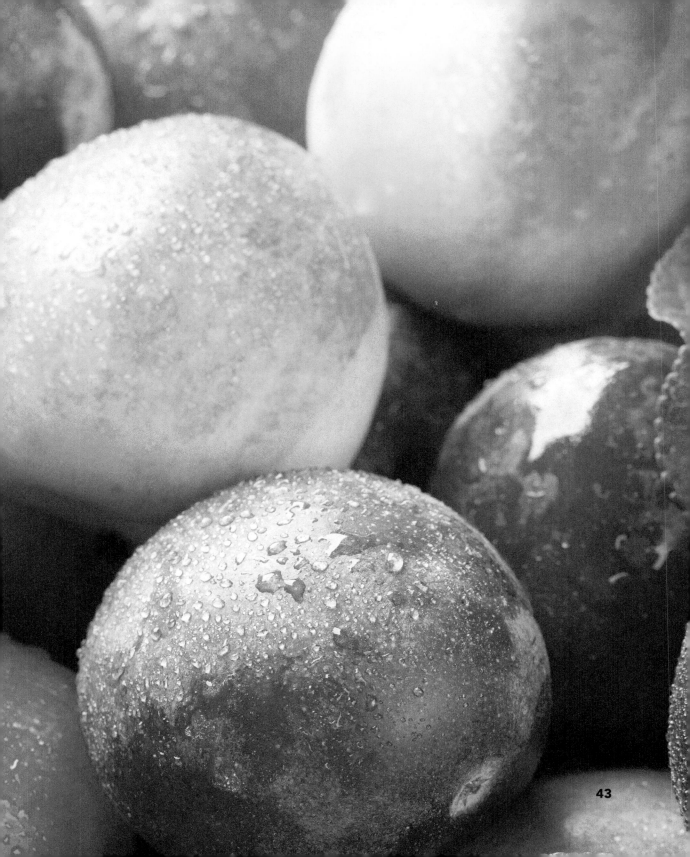

for any uber-health-conscious person. There are plenty of great ready-made options, full of flavour and healthy. Check out brands like Odd pods, Fiid, and Merchant Gourmet for pouches of delicious pulses you can pop in the microwave and serve. I love them with a packet of veg and some flavoured tofu - Tiba Tempeh or Taifun are some of my favourites. Or some lovely chicken or fish.

If you are on the go, try popping into Marks and Spencer's of similar. They do some brilliant takeaway foods. Grab a pot of three bean salad, edamame beans with soy sauce, spiced baked cauliflower, cherry tomatoes filled with feta, some prawns and calamari. Delicious! You may want to grab a ready-cooked chicken breast or cooked mackerel fillet plus a packet of vegetables and a sachet of Merchant lentils in tomato sauce and throw it in the microwave at the office. Nothing wrong with oil or dressings. Food is a privilege and a pleasure; you must eat what you like. No cutting sauces or restricting flavours. Lunch is the main meal of the day because the purpose of eating is energy and power, so around midday or 1pm is your prime time for eating.

Snack

That lunch should fill you up for a while. Still, generally, humans are hungry every four hours and get sugar cravings every two, so it's a good idea always to have a mid-afternoon fruit snack. This is the ideal time for fruit. Fruit is acid, so you don't want to mix it with other foods as it can rot in the belly. Have you noticed how you can get heartburn if you eat fruit for pudding? Avoid mixing fruit with yoghurt, particularly as the acid and alkaline combination is unsuitable for digestion. Additionally, the yoghurt wraps around the fruit, killing off its opportunity to provide much-needed vitamins.

There are hundreds of different types of fruit are out there, and you can enjoy almost all of them. There are only a few that I recommend avoiding because they are very high in fast-acting sugars, more on why that's best avoided later. These few are watermelon, pineapple, melon, banana, kiwi, mango and dried fruits like dates and raisins. We are not naked on a desert island running around eating coconuts all day (sadly!), nor are we jumping around burning energy, eating bananas all day.

Go ahead and snack on apples, peaches, pears, cherries, plums, strawberries and every other delicious fruit you can think of. The possibilities are endless. This is fruit sugar, so you have your weight in kilos in grams of sugar before it even starts to store as fat in your intestine.

Dinner

Having a big meal in the evening is strange. We are most active during the day and need the most energy. During the evening, we are almost always sitting, at a restaurant or in front of the television. So, dinner needs to be a much lighter meal. You've eaten carbohydrates with your seeds, veg, salad, pulses and fruit all day. Dinner can have a carb such as a pulse. Still, logically you mainly need serotonin at night to sleep, so protein is best, plus a pulse for fibre. There is no need to have large amounts of vegetables yet again to wake you up at night.

That might look like steak with a few mushrooms or butter beans, cod served with lentils, trout with capers, tofu with edamame or delicious chicken with cannellini beans. Use lots of lovely herbs and spices, and enjoy sauces with your food. Think Indian food, and there is dal with chicken. Think middle eastern, and there is chicken with hummus. Japanese is often fish and edamame. So those pulses have been around for a very long time.

Years ago, I was vegetarian for 21 years and always had a huge, bloated belly. This was partially caused by eating many vegetables late at night (I was a publisher with Hearst for many years publishing Zest Magazine, the top health and fitness magazine in Europe). I often had late work dinners to attend, a sure-fire way of having a morning belly! Vegetables late at night are challenging for your body to digest whilst sleeping.

Think of your dinner as it would be served in a quality restaurant. You receive the fish, sauce, or pulse you requested when you order. Sides are extra to be ordered. So, think of your portion size as that of a posh restaurant for dinner. Just the middle of the plate and no more. You will be sitting on your bottom for the rest of the night.

You should find it easy to order this meal in good restaurants, so enjoy eating out as often as you want to. This is the standard meal in the best places, and sides are added on extras that you don't have to order. I eat out several times a week, and you can see many of my meals if you follow me on Instagram (@ theweightlossgurucom). They might give you some inspiration.

Eating for life

So, what do you think? Is that something you can do, not just for a week or two, but long term? I never want to see you restricting yourself and picking dejectedly at a flavourless lettuce leaf. So, let's embrace this abundance of delicious food and reclaim the joy of eating for pleasure and health.

The Glycaemic Index

The simplest way to know which foods are the healthiest to eat during your weight management phase is to look at a Glycaemic Index chart. I have attached one on the next page for your perusal.

As I said before, carbohydrates are good, and we must eat them all day. But some carbohydrates could be better during this stage, and these are what I am going to mention here. The GI of a food is the measurement of its load or how it might affect your blood sugar load, so high GI food can cause insulin production, which we want to avoid. For example, the chart shows that the GI of honey is 87, and the GI just below white table sugar (sucrose) is 59.

We don't want anything with a GI like sugar, so let's opt for all carbohydrates with a GI of 40 or below. Luckily almost all of nature's carbohydrates are about 40 or below, so that's easy. Almost all veg – cabbage, kale, broccoli, aubergine, cauliflower- are practically all below 40 or near enough, so that's great. Same with most fruits – blueberries, blackberries, strawberries, pears, apples etc. There are just a few carbohydrates that don't sit under 40, which is often a result of our treatment of them. This chart shows some of the carbohydrates that are not so great in the weight management stage.

Food	Score	Food	Score
Sugars		**Grains & Grain Product**	
Glucose	100	French Baguette	95
Maltose	100	White Rice	72
Honey	87	Bagel	72
Sucrose (Sugar)	59	White Bread	69
Fructose	20	Wholemeal Bread	69
		Ryvita	69
		Crumpet	69
Fruit		Brown Rice	66
Dates	105	Pastry	59
Watermelon	72	Basmati Rice	58
Pineapple	66	Sourdough	54
Melon	65	White Spaghetti	50
Raisins	64	Instant Noodles	46
Banana	62	Wholegrain Wheat Bread	46
Kiwi Fruit	52	Wholegrain Spaghetti	42
Mango	52	Wholegrain Rye Bread	41
Grapes	46		
Oranges	40		
Apple	39	**Pulses**	
Plum	38	Baked Beans	48
Pear	38	Butter Beans	36
Grapefruit	25	Chickpeas	36
Cherries	25	Blackeye Beans	33
		Haricot Beans	31
		Kidney Beans	29
Cereals		Lentils	29
Puffed Rice	80	Red Lentils	16
Cornflakes	67	Soya Beans	15
Muesli	66		
Kelloggs Special K	54		
Kelloggs All Bran	52	**Vegetables**	
Porridge Oats	49	Parsnips (cooked)	97
		Potato (baked)	85
		Cooked Carrots	85
Dairy Products		French Fries	75
Ice Cream	50	Potato (new)	70
Yoghurt	36	Beetroot (cooked)	64
Whole Milk	34	Sweetcorn	59
Skimmed Milk		Sweet Potato	54

If you look at the root vegetables, bottom right on the chart, you can see how crazy high their GI is – 85 for potatoes, 59 for sweetcorn (same as table sugar) and look at parsnips! This is because we don't eat these foods out of the ground raw. We cook them for a long while, the starches caramelise, and then we usually coat them in fat and salt. If we were still farmers, hunters, and gatherers, that would be fine because the energy we expended during the day matches the GI. If we were still living in the agricultural revolution, these foods would have been great for us all day - but that was hundreds of years ago. We were moving all day as labourers, miners, and farmers, so everything was good. Nowadays many people move 2 metres an entire day from their bed to their desk and back again!

Look at the GI chart above for the root vegetables. You can see the incredible pulses - these are superfoods. Low GI, high fibre, very cheap to buy, delicious when cooked correctly, and carb and protein. What's there not to like? You could live on pulses and find it hard to put on weight. We are supposed to have 30 grams of fibre per day. Even with 100 gms of pulses, we only achieve about 8 gms of fibre. Pulses are the superfood.

Now compare that with the grains on the chart. Which of these grains listed has any nutritional value, a GI less than 40 or any key ingredient other than bulking agents such as flour or starch? Starch is a wonderful thing if you need to bulk up with energy all day because of your intensely physically demanding job. But is that you? Or anyone in today's world? That is precisely the problem. Yet the young in the 21st century usually eat about 80% of their food from these grains. So now you're beginning to understand why obesity is becoming an epidemic. I always explain this in terms of culture.

I lived in Asia for 15 years (longer than I've ever lived in London!), and many of my friends and clients are Asian. We could eat rice if we worked in the paddy fields all day. But none of us works in paddy fields. Indeed, most of my Asian clients are bankers in Canary Wharf with almost sedentary jobs.

I also lived in Qatar for a year. I have many Arab friends and clients. None of my Arab clients currently climb desert hills in Qatar. Instead, many of them spend most of their day in their Lamborghini!

If you're from the west, does that mean you have to eat chips, curry, scones and pork pie all day? Absolutely not! We are supposed to eat the way of our lifestyle, not just because of our culture; therefore, it's all going wrong now. Most of the western world is still eating as though we're back in agricultural times with significant energy expenditure every day. That stopped hundreds of years ago for most cultures. If you want a bowl of rice, that's wonderful and up to you. Just remember that a bowl of rice can be up to 8 spoons of processed sugar, so allow an extra two-hour walk in your day for every bowl of rice you choose to have. Is it worth it? Replace these grains with pulses whenever possible, and you'll see the fat pouring off you.

Continue looking at the chart and look at dairy. No animal in the wild suckles a cow apart from a human, which is unnecessary. Lactose is a carb, a fat, and a protein, so it has one purpose only – for babies not yet on food. As soon as you are no longer breastfed, you don't need cow's milk. You can receive all the nutrients you need from the good food you eat.

Looking at the cereals on this chart explains why there has been a tripling of obesity in nursery schools over the last few years. Look at porridge – not much different from table sugar – the porridge oats marketing people really have done a fantastic job! However, it is better than many of the sugary cereals out there.

Then lastly, on this chart, all fruit is good, so I don't bother to list the thousands of good ones because there isn't room. Here at the top, I have listed the few with a GI of significantly over 40. However, I have listed the 7 that could be better here. The tropical fruits and, again – our lifestyle is different from the needs of the past when maybe those fruits kept us alive on a desert island.

A Word About Calories

I don't believe in counting calories. Partly that's because as soon as you start counting calories, you start thinking about restriction. You feel like you can't eat as much as you want to, and your diet is limited. Then you either get obsessive or want to break free, which is no way to spend the rest of your life.

The other reason I will never ask you to count calories is that it doesn't work. Calories are just a measurement of the energy contained in your food. The calorie count doesn't tell you anything about food's health. An avocado contains the same calories as a Creme Egg. Still, the avocado is also full of healthy fats, vitamins and other good things. Likewise, a salmon steak and 9

Jaffa Cakes have the same calorie count. Still, only one is full of protein that will help you build a healthy body and keep you full all afternoon.

Calories only give you part of the story. Health is always the most important thing. When you work towards good health, the weight will fall away. As we said in chapter 2, you can eat more when you increase your skeletal muscle. Start making those changes, and calories won't matter.

It is helpful, however, to know the science behind calories. That way, you will understand why we have the obesity problem in most societies globally, and you will learn how to respond if someone questions you about your eating habits.

Currently, 75% of Americans and just as many British are obese or overweight. That's not all. The problem is steadily growing. By 2030 it's predicted that 50% of the Western Hemisphere will be obese. That is a BMI of 30 or over. The scientific recommendation is a BMI of 18.9 to 24.9. Nearly 6 million of us will be struggling with health conditions such as type 2 diabetes, in the UK, by 2030. This can be prevented if we only spread the word about eating for better health.

If you want to know how many calories you should eat, the easiest thing to do is open your smart scale app and look at your BMR or Basal Metabolic Rate. This is the number of calories you could eat in a day and stay the same weight, plus you can add a few more if you exercise. Then, if you still need to get a smart scale, take your kg weight and multiply it by 30. The theory we always hear is if you want to lose weight, you need to be in calorie deficit. This means you need to eat 500 calories less per day to achieve the 3500 calorie deficit; achieving a 1lb weight loss per week. But, that doesn't allow for the quality of calories, how much you move, how high your skeletal muscle is...

According to the British Medical Journal, we are currently eating an average of about 3500 calories per day per person. An average man eating that much will gain 2 lbs of fat weekly. An average woman, who only needs 1900 calories a day, will gain over 3 lbs of fat per week. So you can see how quickly we get to a situation where most of the population is obese! It is more helpful to know that the average should be about 1900 calories for a woman and 2500 for a man.

The problem with this formula is that it doesn't allow for what calories you are using during your day. For example, standing for 10 hours can use up to 1000 calories. If you get up and do about 20 or 30-minute steady-state cardio in the morning, you can burn up to about 300 calories. Suppose you have high skeletal muscle and low subcutaneous fat. In that case, you can burn about 500 calories in your average day just by moving and the natural chemical reactions your muscles make to use energy.

Suppose we were to stay in bed all day with a hangover. In that case, you could look at our BMR because you're not using any energy, but for most people taking 500 calories off their BMR would leave them almost on a starvation diet – which is another problem with 'diets' – they are all about restrictions which this plan does not do. But, as I said, calories are not the whole story. They are a quick and easy way to keep count but tell us nothing about how healthy a food is.

When I went out for breakfast the other morning, I had some wild mushrooms, harissa beans and scrambled egg. I put that into a calorie counting app, and it informed me I'd had 250 calories. I advise you to steer clear of these supposed 'calorie counting 'apps. Mushrooms with a sauce, harissa beans and scrambled egg (three), probably with butter and cream, as it was a restaurant, in reality, would come in at rocketing 450 calories or more! Since health is the most important thing, that's the last you will hear from me about calories.

The Sugar Roller Coaster

To understand how food affects your health, you must know what happens when you eat. Every time you eat something containing artificial, starchy processed foods, they are broken down by your digestive system and enter your bloodstream as sugar. So whether it's a packet of sweets or wholemeal bread, it doesn't matter. The process is the same. The difference is in the amount of sugar and how quickly it's absorbed.

As the sugar in your blood rises, your body senses it, and your pancreas produces insulin. High blood sugar is life-threatening, and insulin saves your life so your body responds to an emergency. However, your liver and kidneys are in panic mode dealing with this high blood sugar. So how often do animals in the wild eat high-sugar or processed sugar foods?

The insulin unlocks your cells, letting the sugar into your muscles and organs to be used as energy. Any sugar that isn't needed for energy is stored as fat. But, of course, when your blood sugar reaches an average level, your body stops producing insulin, so it never drops too low.

This beautifully designed and carefully balanced system works twenty-four hours a day to keep you healthy. But it can be pushed too far. If you eat a lot of fast-acting processed foods, especially if you constantly snack on high-carb foods, your body produces high insulin levels. Over time, your body may start to become insulin resistant. Those cells become harder to unlock, and your insulin is less effective. So, it would be best to produce more insulin to get the same effect. Eventually, your system can't keep up, and you may be diagnosed with type 2 diabetes.

Even if you don't struggle with insulin resistance, eating fast-acting processed foods still means you are on a sugar roller coaster. First, your blood sugar goes high, giving you a dopamine hit and a rush of energy. But it's a false energy because once that insulin is used to store fat in your cells, you get a blood sugar crash, leaving you tired and reaching for another round of sugars. It's so easy to become addicted to sugar in this way. The more you have, the more you crave!

Non-Alcoholic Fatty Liver disease afflicts 75% of us who are overweight and 90% of us who are obese. The symptoms of this are a bloated belly and water retention. Additionally, you can regularly experience fatigue, your hair could be thinning, and your skin flaky? Does any of this sound familiar?

For every bowl of processed sugar, you need to have that amount again (plus more) of water. One way of measuring it, is that for every 1gram of starch, you need 3grams of water. So, for a 10-mouthful bowl of pasta, you need approximately 30 mouthfuls of water to counteract the water retention. Every time you don't do this, your liver and kidney will struggle. When they rebel, they can start to have fat on them, and they stop working efficiently. You have fat blocking the full function of your organs. The body's response goes on a massive water retention exercise to try and find the water it needs to digest the food now that the liver and kidney can't digest it fully. Remember, a camel's hump is made of fat. As the camel's body is expecting water deprivation for 3 weeks in the desert, it will start storing glucose to compensate for the lack of water. In this way, many humans are willing to create almost a camel's hump on their belly! But again, none of this needs to happen, and it is all reversible. Did you know type 2 diabetes can be reversed within weeks if given the correct help!?

Breaking Sugar Addiction

Many of my clients struggle with sugar addiction, and I'm here to help them break free from that lifestyle. I'm not necessarily talking about sweets and puddings. Even healthy foods like rye bread can contain large amounts of fast-acting sugars. Effectively we are drip-feeding ourselves sugar all day long in our western cultures and not doing the exercise needed to use up all that energy. As a result, most of the western hemisphere live with chronically high levels of insulin, also known as hyperinsulinemia.

The good news is that, unlike a true addiction, your cravings will quickly go when you stop eating so much sugar. This is because you don't really have chemical withdrawal symptoms. It's all about habit. If you don't have sugar for 3 days, it is out of your body. It doesn't own you anymore; therefore, you can longer need it. We will explore emotional eating in chapter 8 since that can be a significant factor. Still, learning which foods will help you improve your health is important.

Don't worry. I'm not about to ask you to give up carbohydrates! This is a very high carbohydrate plan. Carbohydrates make up about 80% of everything we eat - lots of delicious fruits, veg, salad, pulses, spices, herbs and seeds. This is anything but a keto or low-carb diet. Those carbohydrates are incredibly high in water – fruit, veg, salad, spice, and seeds. Hence, they are the natural way you raise your body's water levels, not just through drinking water. Unlike those processed carbohydrates, these natural carbohydrates give you water rather than taking it. I ask you to focus on delicious slow-acting carbohydrates or low GI foods and avoid the ones that give you an unhealthy sugar hit that makes you feel rubbish in the long run.

Protein

Proteins are the building blocks of life. They are used to build muscles, repair your body and even make hormones. Not only that, but they also have no GI, keep you feeling full for ages and are always utilised - lean proteins cannot be stored as fat! Protein is the other most crucial thing to include in your eating lifestyle. You are unlikely to gain weight if you eat lots of the right protein.

Having said that, let's not go to extremes! I am not talking about Atkins or Dukan here, just a healthy diet with lots of healthy protein.

Plant-based Proteins

I recommend that everyone watches "The Game Changers" on Netflix. In it you will discover that many people who demand the most from their bodies, from Roman gladiators to today's top athletes, eat plant-based diets. It's a fascinating documentary. For example, you can see the effect of a single meat-based meal on an athlete's blood. There are also countless stories of athletes breaking records after becoming vegan, and the film shows that a plant-based diet helps with healing and reduces inflammation and the risk of heart disease.

Another thing that you might find interesting is "The China Study", available in bookshops everywhere (including Amazon). This was an extensive study that compared populations all over China and America. They examined which communities had higher rates of a variety of diseases and which lived longer and healthier lives. The most startling conclusion was that the most beneficial populations were the ones that avoided meat, eggs and dairy products.

I'm not asking you to become vegan unless that is something you are already keen to do. It can be a health risk if you don't know what you're doing. Even with all the pulses, you are not getting a complete protein, so B12 injections or supplements might be necessary. Time and again, I have seen things go wrong when people try to restrict themselves and conform to a label. I will not dictate to you. I don't believe in that. The key is finding balance, based on my many years of experience with thousands of clients.

Consider being what I call a "social vegan." Eat plant-based foods much of the time, with lots of excellent carbs/proteins like peas and pulses (chickpeas, red or green lentils, fava beans, black beans, butter beans, cannellini beans, avocado and Tofu). Then, a few times a week have fish, chicken or eggs; with red meat just once a week. This is a really balanced way of eating with a complete protein everyday. The top British heart surgeon, who must be one of the most qualified people to speak on this (1 in 3 people now die of heart-related diseases), recommends a maximum of 70 grams of red meat per week. This is the equivalent of a small piece of steak! Some people are having that twice per day! Top heart surgeons in America now recommend red meat only once per quarter.

You could even start by introducing a "meat-free Monday" or reducing your meat-based meals in another way and go from there. It's not about a label. It's about health. Quorn. Tempeh and Tofu can be excellent replacements but remember they are only a bean. Make sure when you buy them or cook them, they are cooked in a way that makes them delicious, or you won't enjoy them and you'll moan. They need herbs and flavouring like any bean. Why eat the animal that ate the protein when it's healthier to eat protein instead?

Vitamins & Supplements to complement your good foods

If we are eating a healthy lifestyle, then we shouldn't need to take any supplements, powders, or protein bars to achieve a healthy weight and maintain it permanently. There are just a few vitamins suitable to take in the weight loss journey to ensure successful fat loss and energy levels. These are the vitamins that I recommend everyone takes. Our modern lifestyle means that almost everyone can benefit from these. Of course, it's always best to get blood tests if you have symptoms linked to a deficiency. You may need a higher dose, but your doctor will guide you there.

Vitamin D

It's been a long time since we all worked out in the fields in the sun 24/7 or ate raw fish from the river, so for many years, humans have begun losing the ability to convert vitamin D. As much as 50% of the population is deficient in vitamin D and if you spend a lot of time indoors (or outside but well wrapped up against the winter weather!) that almost certainly includes you. If you are vitamin D deficient, then you can't lose fat as vitamin D is the one that holds onto fat, so everyone must take vitamin D in the weight loss stage. When you go to the pharmacy to buy vitamin D3, make sure it also contains K2; without that, it doesn't absorb so well.

<u>This is the product I recommend</u>.

It has both D3 and K2 at the proper doses for most people. There is also a spray available:

<u>You can find it here.</u>

The other thing that nobody ever tells you is that vitamin D is fat-soluble, so you need to take it with food to get the full benefit.

Vitamin C

Why did COVID-19 have such a huge impact? Perhaps because we all have low immune systems. These days our fruit and vegetables aren't grown in the back garden or on a farm down the road. Instead, they are shipped around the world and covered in pesticides. As a result, they can be 75% less nutritious than they used to be. Low vitamin C levels can lead to a weakened immune system and even cancer, so the recommendation is that everyone should take vitamin C. Not only that, if you are deficient in vitamin C (and 50% of us are), then when you exercise, you oxidise 30% less fat than you would if you had normal levels.

<u>This is the Vitamin C that I recommend</u>, at the correct dose for most people.

Vitamin B12

Plant-based proteins are a wonderful thing, but they are not complete proteins. If you choose to eat a vegan diet, I suggest you have blood tests to see if you need B12 injections. Most of my vegan clients have a B12 deficiency, so it's essential to be aware of that possibility and keep yourself healthy.

Turmeric

Turmeric is a natural anti-inflammatory, it's completely harmless, and animals eat it all the time. Still, humans seem to have lost the habit. Studies show you can see huge benefits from eating turmerics such as reducing the chances of dementia, heart disease, depression, cancer, gout, acne, bloating and many more. I especially recommend it for peri-menopausal or menopausal women. As our hormone levels change, our oestrogen levels can dip. With this lack of lubrication, joints may become inflamed, and inflammation can lead to adrenalin, which produces glucose and, therefore, weight gain. Turmeric doesn't work so well on its own, though. It is better when combined with black pepper and ginger. Remember this when you're cooking, you will get some delicious healthy dishes! You can also take supplements that contain all three in perfect quantities. Turmeric is also fat soluble, so it must be taken with food.

This is the one I recommend.

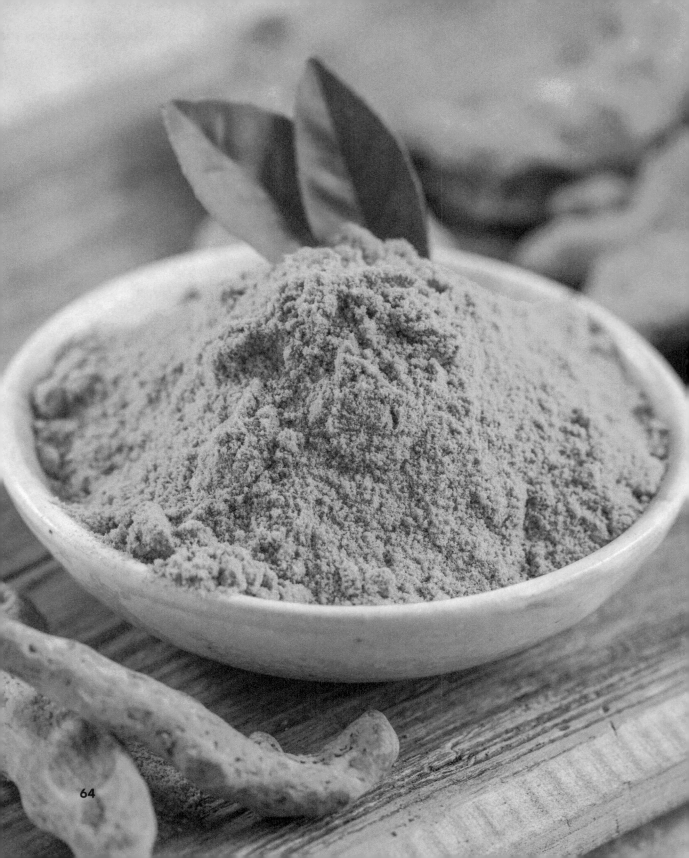

Collagen

The word 'Collagen' comes from a Greek root, or **kolla**, which means "glue." Collagen is the glue that holds us together as we get older. It is the strength and structure of our bodies. Most collagen is found in the connective tissue between our bones, and its loss can result in achy joints. As you may know, our collagen starts to deplete from 20 years old & onwards. So, by the time we're over 40, the lack of it can begin to show. We can't measure how much we have, but when it drops, you may have symptoms such as **joint pain, stiff tendons, or ligaments**. Your muscles may weaken. You could also have papery skin. Years ago, as the Publisher of Zest Magazine (Europe's highest selling Health and Fitness Magazine), I didn't believe collagen could be ingested until I heard about collagen loading. If you load up with collagen for a month when you first start taking it, you have much better chance of replacing your younger age levels faster and thereafter maintaining them. I consume a sachet of collagen daily, having already done some collagen loading. So, whether you're male or female, once you are over 35, I recommend you start looking for a good one.

Probiotics

I sometimes hear people say they "take a probiotic", but it's impossible to know which one you might need. Probiotics are so varied. There are hundreds of them! It's like saying you need an antibiotic; you need to be more specific. That's why I only recommend probiotic pills if you have been analysed. Instead, get your probiotics from natural sources, which give you variety and often taste delicious. Lovely things like Kafir, Kombucha, Kimchi and Sauerkraut are easy to add to your diet and give you the probiotics you need. Don't forget your Greek yoghurt and plant-based yoghurt are also good sources of probiotics – good gut health.

Yasmin, David and Sophie

Yasmin

Yasmin thought she was eating well, but now she realised she was consuming a lot of sugar without realising it.

She will be ditching her snacks of dried fruits and granola bars and throwing an apple or pear in her bag instead. Yasmin won't have her rye bread sandwiches or sushi for lunch anymore. She plans to enjoy all her favourite fillings as big salads instead – humus, dal, chicken, tuna and eggs mixed with edamame, avocado, lentils, rocket and maybe even feta to make it even more delicious. Olive oil and balsamic vinegar dressing too. It's so great not to feel restricted.

David

David has been relying on processed foods and takeaways as a busy person living alone. But, unfortunately, his favourite pizza, smothered in gooey cheese, isn't doing his health any good!

He is going to pick up some of the ready-made options. Today he had a salmon fillet with a pouch of delicious chickpea tagine and a large bag of mixed vegetables cooked in the microwave. Great for a meal that only took a few minutes in the microwave!

Sophie

Sophie's husband has been watching a lot about how to be leaner and fitter to reduce belly fat. He can see vegan options as one way to become less 'flesh' focused. He's also been reading about climate change recently. He has been talking about going vegan to reduce his carbon footprint too. Having watched "The Game Changers" together, they plan to include more plant-based meals, starting with three nights a week and building up from there.

Having always grabbed toast for breakfast and a quick sandwich for lunch, usually on the go, sitting down to eat a meal feels a little daunting. Sophie even felt self-conscious sitting at the table on her own to eat lunch, as if she should be rushing off to do a chore instead of eating. So she will stick with it for now and explore it a little further in chapter 8.

Over to You

Are you ready to get started with your new lifestyle? Take a few minutes to get out your iPhone notes or journal and think through your plans for the next few days. Then make a shopping list that will set you up for success.

You should read chapter 4 before you start, but if you don't want to wait, you can make more changes as you go along.

Remember, there are no rules on this program. When you start, just one bowl of pasta less per week might make a difference for some people. One night refraining from alcohol per week might be progress. All these are baby steps, but whatever changes you are comfortable with. Every single step is a step towards improving or even saving your life. One better decision each day will eventually become a complete life change. Some of my clients start with two better weekly choices about food and alcohol, and three months later, they have lost three stones, and they are saying how easy it was to make the right changes. This is not a challenge, this is not scary, and there is no pressure. If you are overwhelmed by giving up pasta, bread and potatoes altogether, consider how you could take a step in that direction. Could you have one or two sugar-free days a week? Halve your serving of sugars and increase the pulses instead? Take one action this week, and then review and see what else you can do next week.

Here are a few prompts for you to think about as you journal.

My Thoughts on Food for This Week

Will I be at home or out and about over the next few days?

Do I have the time and inclination to cook, or are ready-made options better?

Are there any social events that I need to consider?

Do I have any other goals, such as including vegan meals?

My top three breakfast ideas (restaurant-sized and protein-based)

My top three lunch ideas (double protein, restaurant-sized plus!)

My favourite fruits to snack on, avoiding watermelon, pineapple, melon, banana, kiwi, mango and dried fruits.

My top three lighter dinners

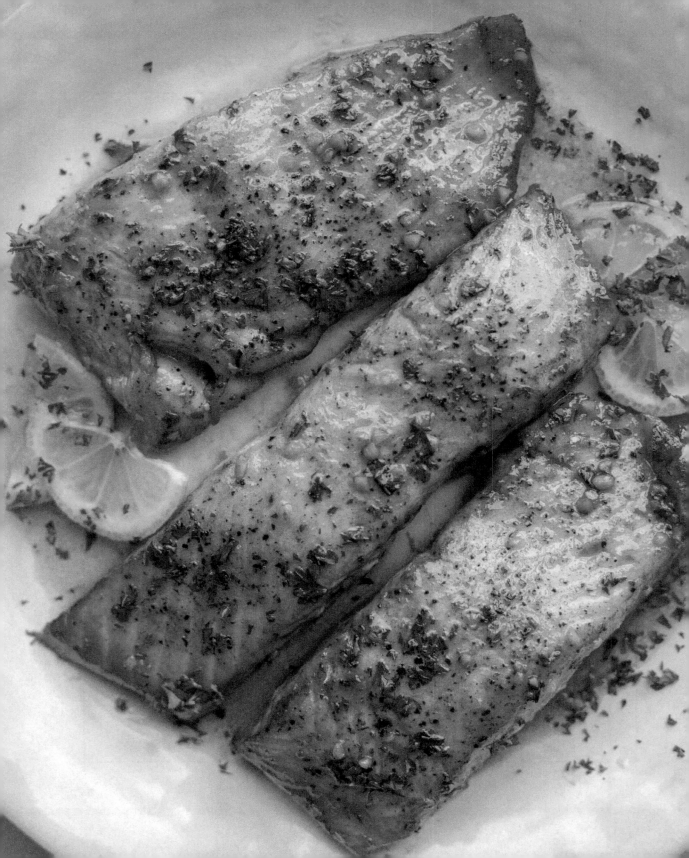

E - Eating Times for Modern Lifestyles

"Eating After 8 PM is Worst Time of Day to Eat for Weight Loss."
- Margaret Davis Science Times

Do you believe in a traditional way of eating? Most people do. It seems ingrained into our culture. We tend to eat soon after we wake up, grabbing a coffee and something quick as we race out the door and probably feeling guilty that we didn't have a "proper breakfast". Lunch might be grabbed at your desk at 12 or 1. Dinner is the main meal and is served in the evening, at 8pm. Of course, there are exceptions, weekend brunches and afternoon teas or a Sunday roast served at lunchtime. Still, those are perceived as 'treats' and made more special by being different.

That's how it always is in every TV show or advert, every meal planning booklet or menu. It's how meals have been structured throughout history, biologically necessary and part of being human. Isn't it?

Actually, it's not.

This "traditional" way of eating has only been around for a very short time since sugar was invented, and really, it's a bit weird. This chapter will explore natural meal timings that make sense and support your health and modern lifestyle.

What time is dinner?

That is a surprisingly exciting and complex question! Humans have been around for about 150,000 years, and we have lived by the sun for much of that time.

Everyone followed a roughly similar pattern for thousands of years, from cave dwellers to farmers and monks. First, we would wake up early and head off to exercise, perhaps gathering, hunting, or working in the fields. Then we would eat breakfast. Then, after some more activity, everyone would eat a big meal in the middle of the day, the perfect opportunity to fuel our bodies for the afternoon. Food was a daytime need, and people ate when they needed energy.

By early evening it's starting to get dark, so people have gathered in caves, huts or houses. This occurred for thousands of years. They would batten down the hatches, share stories and songs, rest and sleep. This was not the time when anyone would set off hunting or start the hours-long process of cooking over a fire, especially with no light. Nobody needed food, as they weren't doing anything to burn energy.

Isn't it a bit weird to think of a farmer, hunter, or gatherer suddenly jumping up at 8pm and heading off into the dark to go hunting? Can you imagine a lion suddenly killing an animal to eat it late at night? It makes no sense to wake yourself up by eating late in the evening.

The modern habit of eating late started very recently, in the blink of an eye, in human history. It is anything but normal or natural. It is normal to eat your biggest meal in the middle of the day – lunch and eat little or nothing after about 5 or 6pm.

Even if you look back at photos of the 1970s, almost everyone looks slim. Even in an era when they didn't always have the most nutritious food, most people stayed a healthy weight. Why? Because they ate dinner early.

The One Thing that Makes the Biggest Difference

Whenever I ask my successful clients what made the most significant difference to their weight loss journey, they say that changing their dinner time had a considerable impact.

The Times newspaper did a feature on this, where they said that if you eat at 8pm, you are on a death wish. Dramatic wording but not too far from the truth. That's because it takes four hours for your food to be digested and even longer to work it off. So if you eat at 8pm and go to bed at 10 or 11, your food hasn't even reached your stomach.

Your body is full of energy, fuelled, and ready to run a marathon, but instead, you get into bed. Now you have a conflict. Your head wants to sleep while your body is wide awake. So you toss and turn all night, not getting the rest you need, and the only option your body has is to send in lots of insulin and store all that energy as fat. Most people never really enjoy the nutritional benefits of their dinner. It gets stored as fat. If you have a big belly, then this is most likely the reason.

What is the alternative if eating at 8pm is so bad for your health? As I said, it takes about four hours to digest a meal, so humans get hungry roughly every four hours. But we can get a sugar dip every two hours so a fruit snack is always a good option around 3pm or 4pm to keep you going till you're genuinely hungry around 6pm for dinner. So, if you have lunch at around 12 or 1, you will be hungry at 4 or 5. Have you ever heard people say you should never schedule a 4pm meeting? This is a big reason that everyone is exhausted; by 5pm, they are starving! So, what do we do? Most people turn to biscuits or cake to "keep them going", or they have an alcoholic drink. It raises your sugars and gives you energy, but it's temporary. By 8pm, you are absolutely starving because you haven't eaten since lunch, so you eat a huge meal, and it's all sitting in your stomach when you go to bed.

What if you listened to your hunger and ate dinner early? Food is for life, for energy. A daytime need, not evening greed. Food is your fuel, and at 6pm, you are running on empty - so doesn't it make sense to refuel? Then you would be ready for the next part of your day. You could work later if you wanted to without feeling burnt out or go to the gym without feeling exhausted. You could see friends or spend time with your family, feeling confident, happy and free from any pressure to cook! Then, after a fun evening doing the things you enjoy, you will naturally feel tired at bedtime. You'll even find that you sleep much better and wake up feeling refreshed and full of energy, with a flat belly instead of a fat one.

But what about:

A 6pm dinner time is unusual these days, but isn't it worth a try for your health? Of course, we all have obstacles to overcome, but it is possible with some thought and willingness to try.

… my job?

Many of my clients are at work at 6pm, but usually, they can take a break and eat dinner. Even if that means moving a few other things around or having a shorter lunch. These days many employers are more concerned about results than the number of hours you spend at your desk anyway, so they will be delighted if you boost your productivity for the rest of the afternoon! As we said in the last chapter, dinner is smaller, so it will take a little time to eat anyway.

… my partner?

This can be a bit trickier, but most of us have spouses or partners who are used to having dinner in the evening. Remember that what they choose to do may work well for them. Perhaps they are taller than you or have a different metabolism. However, it is not working for you, and you are entitled to make that change for your health. If they love you, then surely, they want you to be healthy and will support you? You can still sit with them at 8pm and be charming and eloquent while they eat. You can save a portion of their dinner for your lunch the next day - a great way to cut down on cooking.

... my social life?

Do you eat out a lot? I do, and many of my clients do as well! Eating out can be a wonderful part of your new lifestyle, so don't feel you need to give it up. In the initial weight loss phase, stick to an early dinner as often as possible, but if you are eating late in a restaurant you still have plenty of options. Choose a protein dish, perhaps fish or chicken, and avoid adding a sugary side like rice or potatoes. If you eat early Sunday to Wednesday and then later other evenings, you will still have significantly improved your health.

If you want to socialise without eating always being the focus, you could suggest doing something else. For example, going to the theatre or cinema, walking around the lake, dancing or joining a choir, attending an art class together or just going for a walk. There are so many possibilities.

... my late bedtime?

Only some people go to bed at 10 or 11pm, and clients sometimes ask me if they can eat at 8pm since they only go to bed at 1am, well over the four-hour threshold.

Unfortunately, it doesn't work that way. If you eat at 6pm or earlier, you will move around after your meal. Commuting home from work, playing with your children, going for an evening stroll. Even just getting things done around the house. That activity uses up the energy from your meal. So what are you doing between 9pm and 1am? Almost certainly sitting still, either watching TV or working at a computer. It just isn't the same.

Are you sure you are hungry? Think about it. You would not feed a pet at 11pm. You wouldn't give a five-year-old a biscuit or cook a meal if they got out of bed in the middle of the night. We know that these things wouldn't be healthy. So, if you wouldn't make a dog unwell by feeding it biscuits late in the evening, don't do the same thing to yourself. You deserve to respect, love and care for yourself at least as much as you care for the family pet, surely?!

Go to Chapter 8 (Investigate) to determine whether you are hungry and find out what to do about it.

Autophagy

I only encourage going vegan if it is something you want to do (as it can be too limiting), nor do I endorse fasting on this plan. Again, unless it's something you want to do for health reasons. My way is intermittent eating, not intermittent fasting. We are not timing when we eat. Eating dinner at least 4 hours before bed makes sense so your food reaches your belly and breakfast approximately 2 hours after you wake up to use up some fat-burning time. However, this is no denying that in practically every culture since time began, there has been some element of fasting or cell renewal practice.

Many years ago, humans used to live to around 40, and we have now doubled that life expectancy. Imagine if we could double it again and live to be 150 or more! Wouldn't it be wonderful to think that you still had so much of your life to live? The truth is that we don't die of old age. We pass away due to the complications associated with old age. Avoid those complications, and we can live for as long as we want!

Currently, one in two of us will get cancer. One in three will die of a heart-related condition. In addition, as we age, we sometimes get arthritis, Alzheimer's and various eye conditions, all of which can be reversed or avoided by cell renewal.

Autophagy is like rebooting your computer, but for your body. It allows your body to switch off and renew so that you feel full of energy, with everything from your cells to your nerve endings firing like new. It's an empowering feeling. So, how do you make it happen? The truth is that if you constantly drip-feed your cells with sugar (as most people do), they never have a chance to renew. It's only when you have a break from eating that any form of autophagy has a chance to happen. Having a break from food from, say, 6pm until 10am is almost like rebooting your computer, but this is your body. You can reboot your cells by turning them off and then back on again if you pause from food for 12 hours or more.

My mother died of cancer, so autophagy is something that I have been interested in for a long time. I would never say that it can prevent or cure cancer. Of course, you must also listen to doctors and have other treatments. But it is scientifically proven, without a doubt, to make a big difference. This is about health first and foremost; weight loss is a handy side effect.

Real autophagy kicks in when you fast for 48-72 hours, which is quite extreme. Many people fighting cancer choose to go down this route, and I completely respect that decision. It's up to you if you want to try it, but it's unnecessary for the health and weight loss we are talking about.

A 72-hour fast certainly gives you an incredible boost of energy, it's a fantastic thing to experience, but that would be something for you to research elsewhere if you're interested in trying it. The good news is that even a short fast of 16 hours overnight is enough to have some autophagy, making a real difference to your health.

When you eat dinner early and breakfast late, your body starts to run like a Tesla. Just like a computer, you can reboot your system. As a result, you wake up each morning well-rested and full of energy, excited to start your day. Doesn't that sound amazing?

You will not get these benefits if you have dinner at 8pm, breakfast at 6am, or even 7pm and 7am. It would help if you gave your body a chance to rest and renew, so we aim for 16 hours between dinner and breakfast. But remember, this is not about intermittent fasting, so don't worry about the numbers. This is intermittent eating; a late breakfast and an early dinner are all you need. But remember the most important meal is always this big lunch at midday.

Lunch

So, remember that the day's main meal must always be lunch. Breakfast and lunch should be significant, think pub grub size plus more for lunch. We are on this planet to work, whether at home, in the office or outside, and midday is the most critical time of the day to give yourself energy. Humans have been around 150,000 years, and for the first 149,000, we were in bed when dark, at 5pm. We were energised farmers, hunters, gatherers, and labourers all day. So, we know eating in the evening in today's lifestyle can not work. So, lunch must be the big boy!

Which Plan Works for You?

This is about crafting a lifestyle that works for you, with eating times that support your health. Of course, you know yourself best, so I can't and won't give you specific mealtimes to follow. Instead, I will provide you with three examples, and you can see which would be the best fit. Try out all three, give each one a week, and then make your decision.

Breakfast

You will notice that, as well as an early dinner, these examples all include a late breakfast. That's because when you wake up in the morning, your cortisol level is low, your blood sugar is low, and your body has no choice but to burn fat for energy. Exercising before eating is the best way to burn visceral fat. You are "in the shred". However, you do have to eat at some point during the morning to kick-start your metabolism and burn calories. So don't try to skip breakfast altogether! Particularly over the age of 40. My clients of that age or over who skip breakfast start putting on weight. At that age, our body is not so adaptable. If you don't eat all morning, you could be listless and under-energised when you should be doing some good work. Also, when your body suspects there might be a lack of food around for some reason (like winter in the wild for animals), it might switch off to conserve energy for the lean times ahead (like hibernation). And it could even lead to weight gain.

Schedules

Please remember that although I'm giving specific times, this is not a diet or a restrictive plan. You don't have to set the alarm, eat at the exact times stated, or sit with a growling stomach as you watch the minute hand creep around.

There are no rules. These examples help you to apply the principles. For instance, I can't eat breakfast any later than 9, but that's OK. But to start with, try aiming for these times. If you are hungry less than four hours after a meal, it is likely a craving rather than actual hunger. You can find more information on cravings in chapter 8.

Option 1 – the standard plan

This is the closest to the meals you are probably used to, which makes it the most straightforward plan to start with:

10am - big breakfast
1pm - huge lunch
3pm – fruit snack

6pm - light dinner

If you get very hungry before 10am, please have breakfast earlier. You may start your day at 5 and need breakfast by 7! Remember that this plan is only a guide and not a rule. For example, suppose you generally try to have breakfast approximately two hours after you wake up. In that case, you'll have plenty of time to burn fat before eating.

Option 2 – fat loss boost

This way of eating is great if you want to boost your weight loss or if you find (as many people do) that option 1 feels like a lot of food. You will notice that it's also incredibly similar to the way we ate for centuries. This shows us that it is a natural and comfortable way to eat once you get used to the change; it's also how many elite athletes eat. This fits better with your lifestyle, especially if you work in an office where taking time out for three meals could be tricky. By not eating between 5pm and 11am, you are giving yourself a weight loss boost every time.

11am - early, hearty lunch (call it brunch if you like, but eat lunch foods)
3pm - fruit platter
4pm - dinner

Option 3 – fruit dinner plan

After a week or so of eating this way, many of my clients say that they aren't very hungry in the evening. This is because they have a big breakfast and a huge lunch; some days, they don't want dinner. This is where the fruit dinner is a fantastic thing to add to your toolbox.

Prepare a big platter of fruit. Perhaps strawberries, nectarines, apple slices and blueberries. Whatever your favourites are, pile your plate high. Just avoid the seven high-sugar fruits. Instead, try and eat with the seasons – winter might be 5 pieces of fruit such as pears, apples, satsumas, or plums. Summer might be 3 packets of fruit such as strawberries, raspberries and peaches.

When you feel hungry, say between 2.30 and 6.30, graze from your fruit platter, and it will fill you up. You can even eat it while you sit at your desk, so this works brilliantly for busy people. The fruit will be enough, so you won't need anything else until breakfast the next day. You can spend your evening chatting with your family or enjoying a hobby instead of cooking.

Often my clients find that they lose a lot of fat when they try this, perhaps as much as 1lb a day. This makes it a helpful tactic if you know you have eaten more than you usually would and the weight is starting to creep on. For example, if you have a weekend away and enjoy several big evening meals, have a few days with fruit dinners when you get home, and you'll be back on track. Finding the balance is easy, and nothing needs to be off-limits.

Please don't get scared by this option. If it sounds too extreme, stick with options 1 and 2, and you will lose weight. The results of having a huge breakfast and lunch and then grazing on fruit all afternoon and early evening are outstanding, though. You could do this Sunday, Monday, and Tuesday so you feel back on track by Wednesday after an overindulgent weekend. My clients that make the fruit dinner very regularly achieve crazy good results. You can use this plan for a few days to get back on track if you've had an indulgent weekend or several late-evening meals. Alternatively, do this as often as you can.

On the nights you are eating out, if you've already eaten your fruit dinner, no matter how late you start to eat when socialising, you will still make better food choices.

10am - good breakfast
12:30pm - large lunch
3pm - 6pm - graze constantly on delicious fruit

Yasmin, David and Sophie

Yasmin

At first, Yasmin didn't see how she could make this work. Her job finishes at 5pm, so she needed help to get home, cook and eat dinner by 6pm, and breakfast and lunch, all in the 9-5 timeframe. Furthermore, her supervisor was going only to allow so many meal breaks!

With some creative thinking, Yasmin has decided to choose option 2. Her supervisor is happy for her to have a lunch break at 11am instead of noon (she was delighted since now Yasmin can cover her colleague's lunch breaks). So Yasmin will have something hot for lunch, and a pre-cooked dinner will be waiting at home for her to eat as soon as she gets in.

David

Working shifts means that Dave's mealtimes are always a bit hit and miss, and you can only stop for a big, cooked meal when you're out in the ambulance. So he has decided to give Option 3 a try.

Whatever time his shift starts, David will wake a few hours earlier to exercise before breakfast. Fitting in one meal should be doable, and snacking on fruit is much easier than trying to find time for another meal. He is very much looking forward to the autophagy energy boost. As a lifelong insomniac, he's curious to see if eating earlier helps him sleep better.

Sophie

An early dinner is fine for Sophie since it just means eating with the children at 5pm. Although her husband isn't keen on eating alone, she is committed to trying it.

She has decided to try each option for a week to compare how she feels and the results she gets from each. Sophie is quite excited about having the chance to experiment and craft an eating pattern that works for her.

Your Turn

Now is your chance to get out your phone or journal and make some plans. So here are some things you might want to think about:

My first thoughts on eating times

Will I face any challenges?

How can I overcome them?

Trying the Different Options
(Do this for each one individually)

My Smart Scale readings before:

My readings after:

Weight lost:

How I feel:

What went well?

Any logistical or other challenges?

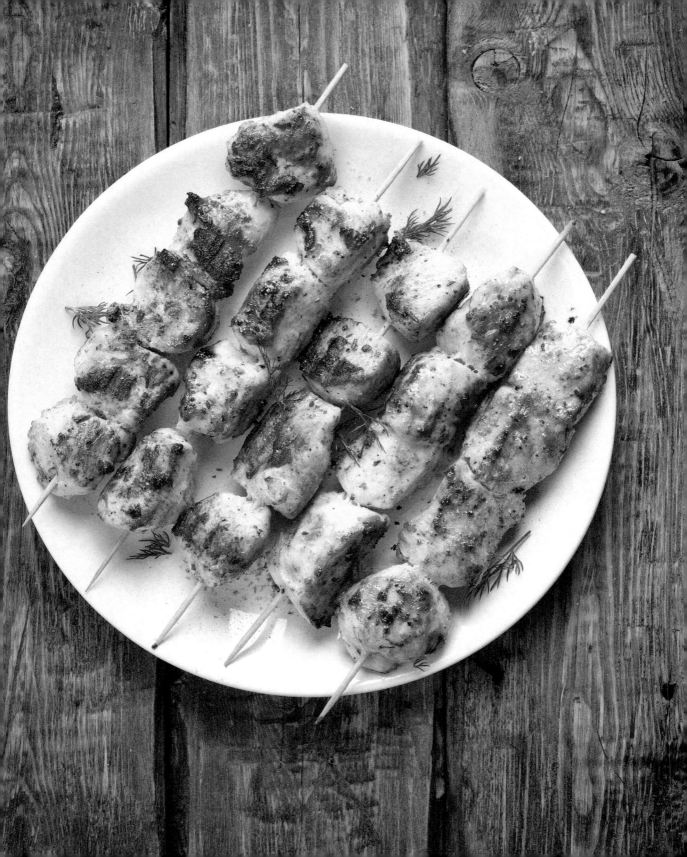

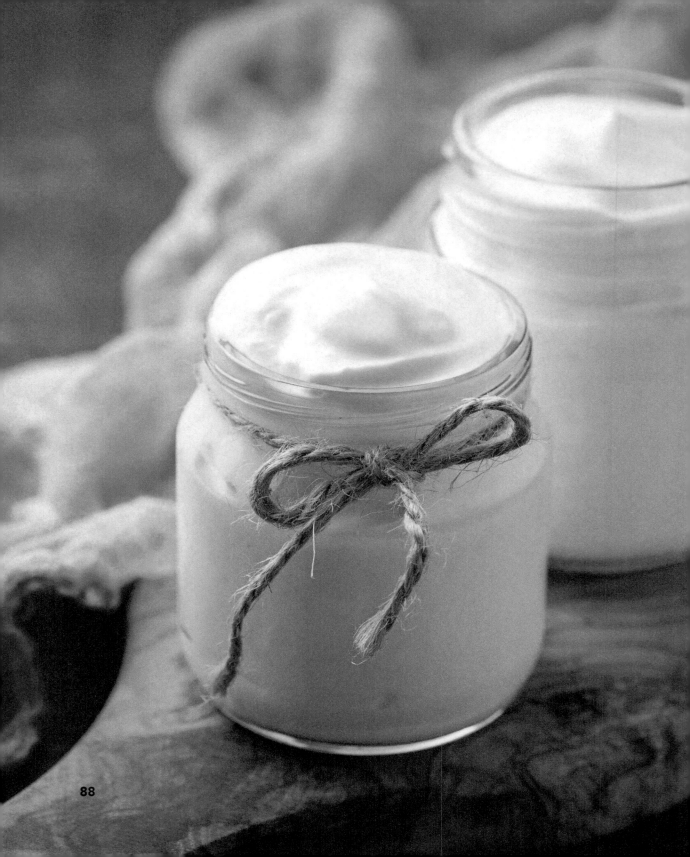

C - Cut the Junk

"Every living cell in your body is made from the food you eat. If you consistently eat junk food then you'll have a junk body."
- Jeanette Jenkins

I don't believe that junk food exists. There is only food - something that nourishes your body supports your health and gives you energy for life - or junk. It can't be both, so "junk food" is a misnomer. You are not a rubbish bin. Filling yourself with rubbish or junk is not going to serve you well. In this chapter, I will help you see how to plan meals that cut out the junk, focusing on the foods that will help you reach your goals and reclaim your healthy, happy life.

We will also do some troubleshooting in this chapter. If you have put all the advice in the previous chapters into practice and are still waiting to see the results you want, you may find something here that will help. There are no rules, which is true. Still, if I were working with you in person, I would be able to offer suggestions and help you make tweaks to discover the exact formula that works best for you. As I can't do that in a book, I will offer various tips and ideas. Please, don't feel you are expected to follow them all rigidly. If you did that, you would end up with a very restricted diet - not our aim! Instead, pick one that seems to resonate with you, try it out and see what happens. Experiment and discover your own perfect mix.

Meal Planning Suggestions

This is not a restrictive "diet", and you will eat plenty of carbohydrates, fats and proteins. This is a high carbohydrate, high protein and high-fat plan. Most of my clients complain they are too full. You are bingeing on carbohydrates daily – fruit, veg, salad, spice, seeds and pulses. You are eating masses of protein all day – Greek yoghurts, fish, lean meat, pulses, eggs, hemp seeds, tofu, avocado, peas etc. You are eating most of the fats you like within reason – olive oil, fish, sauces, and eggs all contain fats. There are so many lovely things you can eat. Imagine feasting on scrambled eggs and smoked salmon for breakfast. What about a tuna, avocado, feta, rocket, and warm chickpea salad sprinkled with pumpkin seeds or chicken served with butter beans and a big pile of roasted vegetables for lunch? Teatime is some fruit, and then for dinner, you have a beautiful seabass with lemon sauce and lentils or capers.

This is not about deprivation and not about following a strict plan either. I don't want you to force down foods you don't like just because I suggested them! But I know it can be challenging to see how to put meals together, so here are some ideas to help you.

Would you go to a lovely restaurant and order toast? You probably wouldn't! Processed, artificial starches like bread, pasta, cereal, biscuits, and cakes are just sugary fillers. Don't see them as carbohydrates. Instead, see them as processed food. You might need that bulk if you are a labourer working in the fields, an elite athlete, or even a growing child. But the average adult in this century doesn't burn off enough energy to need those foods. So cut out the junk and enjoy eating the most delicious food you have ever eaten!

Breakfast

As I'm sure you remember, breakfast is all about protein, which feeds your brain and nurtures your muscles. If you start the day with sugars such as toast or cereal, you've already triggered your dopamine responders to hit an insulin high and crave those kinds of sugars all day. So, think protein. There are many excellent traditional options here, yoghurt, of course, but also things like eggs, kippers, mushrooms, tofu scrambled or avocado. You can even move away from traditional breakfast foods. No rule says you can't have salmon or chicken for breakfast if you want to! Here are a few breakfast suggestions:

Eggs, smoked salmon, plain omelette, avocado, mushroom omelette, kippers, haddock, Greek yoghurt, protein yoghurt, mushrooms, chicken, mung bean porridge, chia pot with almond milk, scrambled tofu, Turkey bacon.

Lunch

Remember, carbohydrates give you energy. You need plenty of energy during the day so eat lots of carbohydrates - vegetables, pulses and so on, especially at lunchtime. Always eat fruit on its own as it is an acid with a very low GI if eaten on its own. Once mixed with alkaline, you can get bloating or rotting fruit in your belly, so fruit is always your afternoon snack. This is when you need lots of energy so be sure to fill it up! This is not a low-carb diet; you need to eat lots of carbohydrates. Just avoid the junk - sugar that does you more harm than good.

Replace the traditional sugars of your meal with extra carbs/protein, usually pulses. So instead of bread, potatoes or pasta, you have lentils, beans or chickpeas. For example, you might have curry but replace the rice with dhal, or have an extra portion of Bolognese sauce plus kidney beans with vegetables but leave the pasta. It's easy to adapt a lot of your usual meals that way. For example, if you love sandwiches, you could make your favourite fillings into salads. Make sure you have plenty of protein to go with the vegetables and serve hummus or edamame beans.

Dinner

By the end of the day, your needs have shifted. It's doubtful that you are about to go and run a marathon. Most of us spend the evening sitting on our bottoms, whether in front of a TV or at a dinner party. You want to feel restful and ready for a good night's sleep in a few hours. So you need foods rich in selenium, in other words, protein foods. Plus, a small number of carbohydrates for fibre – a pulse.

Remember that a dish is just the protein in all the best restaurants when you eat out. Any sides must be ordered as extras, so you can easily choose not to order them! You can apply this principle at home, too. For example, suppose your family is tucking into teriyaki salmon with noodles. In that case, you can have the salmon with some lentils and skip the noodles.

Changing starches for pulses

When your family has a roast at lunchtime, you'll all eat the same, but you will have more roast chicken, vegetables, and maybe some nice butterbeans in the gravy. The kids or someone there who has a physically demanding job might have the roast potatoes to bulk. Their plate will have up to 1000 calories more than yours, but you will feel more satiated as you avoid the sugars. If they have a chicken tikka masala with dal for lunch, you will also have loads of veg to make it more filling. Again, they might have it with rice or naan to bulk.

Fruit snack

Always remember your fruit snack anytime you are hungry between lunch and dinner as you need to keep your energy levels up, and fruit is a fantastic healthy snack, full of fibre when eaten on its own. Just remember that you are avoiding tropical fruits in the weight management phase.

Insulin

Just a reminder of your body's process when you eat starchy processed carbohydrates if you haven't moved much in a day. Potatoes and rice come under this category, too, because although they both come from the ground, they are treated in such a way that they become more starch based. You never eat a potato straight from the ground, do you? It's been cooked for quite a while when the starch caramelises yet further in the cooking process, and then we roast it in fat and mix it with butter and salt. So it is never just a potato. That's why a raw carrot has a GI of 52, whereas a cooked carrot has a GI of 85.

When you eat your bowl of pasta, let's say it's 10 mouthfuls of starch. As you know, 1gram of starch needs 3 mouthfuls of water to digest. That's why natural carbohydrates – fruit, veg, salad, spice, seeds, herbs and pulses are so great as they are full of water. Not so for the processed grains. You have your 10 mouthfuls of pasta, but then you need 30 mouthfuls of water to digest it. That is unlikely to happen, of course. So, your liver is like – I can't do this and starts to dump toxins. Once your liver has fat on, it functions even less efficiently, so your metabolism slows even more. Without that required water, your body has to go into water retention mode, so bloating may start. You might not notice how much you bloat after each bowl of pasta until you stop having so much.

Smokers don't realise how strong cigarettes are until they are non-smokers. All this extra glucose you have gained from this pasta needs to be worked off, but you don't. Your body quickly squirts out insulin to deal with this excess sugar. That insulin grabs all the extra energy and stores it around your middle area as fat. Then you get that insulin dip as you've had the high of the release and then the low as it starts its storing process. Then you feel exhausted and want sleep, or you will have to eat more starches to begin the process again. Wouldn't it have been easier just to have had a delicious plate of pulses, fish and veggies in the first place and avoided this whole process?

Good gut health

With healthy eating, such as I recommend in my program, almost all gut intolerances can be sorted, usually within weeks. If you twist your ankle or knee, it becomes hot to tell you that it is inflamed and needs help. Your gut doesn't have this simple message system, so when it is inflamed, it will send you other messages such as bloating, intolerances, IBS, wind and many others. Follow my plan, and these symptoms will dissipate, if not vanish completely – we are blessed!

The fantastic advantage of cutting junk (in addition to the weight loss) is how quickly it can reverse the symptoms of many commonplace illnesses and issues that my clients, when first starting with me, now so often seem to have. Issues such as IBS (Irritable bowel syndrome), NAFLD (Non-Alcoholic Fatty Liver Disease), SIBO (Small Intestine Bacteria), SIFO (Small intestine fungal disease), gout, bloating, wind, headaches, anxiety, allergens, raised bad cholesterol levels, to name but a few of the many afflictions caused by our current poor gut health.

As good gut health means having more good bacteria than harmful bacteria, it makes sense that excess harmful bacteria often cause poor gut health. This imbalance can occur as a result of antibiotics or food poisoning. However, although these causes can quickly change the balance of bacteria in your gut, an overindulgence in eating junk and gas-forming carbohydrates like the ones mentioned earlier are usually the cause of long-term gut issues and intolerances. For many of my clients, their bloating and/or IBS symptoms disappear almost within weeks of eating on my healthy lifestyle program. Creating and maintaining good gut health can reduce it further until we see an end to these negative symptoms.

We are familiar with the gut's role in digestion, breaking down the food we eat, absorbing the parts we need and disposing of the rest. The pancreas and liver help the gut along in these efforts. The gut is also home to a host of friendly bacteria, which further aid digestion. These good bacteria make up the gut flora, particularly in the colon. Unfortunately, they are also joined by some common species of harmful bacteria. A healthy gut means that there are more good bacteria than harmful bacteria and that harmful bacteria don't overtake the good.

If your gut is healthy, you can imagine it will look like a glorious, luscious, rich Amazon Forest with trees and foliage and new plants and growth everywhere. In that situation, if you were to get ill, the rest of the body can call on the gut saying – help me- and your gut will say, "Yes, I can help you. I'm here for you". So whatever illness you get, you hope you've got excess reserves to fix it.

However, imagine that your gut lacks good bacteria through poor eating, fizzy drinks, and too many antibiotics or medications. Your gut is like a dry, deadwood forest with no excess reserves, no luscious new growth, and no mass of lovely healthy bacteria. When that happens, if we get ill, there are no excess reserves to call on. Your gut will literally say to hold on a minute. There is nothing spare to give. We can not cure ourselves simply in this instance. That is why our gut health is so essential on this health journey. The weight falls off because of healthy eating.

When the balance of bacteria in the gut flora is good, it can lead to many other health benefits, including reducing inflammation that can lead to heart disease and lowering the chance of obesity, reducing the chances of certain cancers, arthritis, dementia, eczema, arthritis etc. So cutting out the junk can save your life and give you the goal body you've always dreamed of having!!

Remember, it takes 4 hours for food to get from the mouth to the belly, so a good measure to test if something you've digested is an allergy or intolerance is how long it takes to show effect. For example, suppose you feel something within just 2 hours of eating. In that case, it is very likely to be an allergy, as it won't have even reached your belly by then for you to start having an intolerance.

Meal plans and recipes included.

As you know, this healthy eating lifestyle is not a 'thing'. It is just eating breakfast later, a large lunch, eating dinner earlier and having fruit as your snack. How simple is that? Nothing complicated and with no rules to follow. So sometimes I almost want to resist giving people all the lovely meal plans, food plans and recipes I provide because they can feel that they must stick precisely to the plan, which is never the idea.

Please do not follow my food plans as prescriptive. Please use them as a guide to delicious food choices. So, you can eat as much as you like during the day of all the good stuff. Just avoid the starchy carbs, and you'll be fine. My food and menu plans are just a guide – not to be followed to the letter. I want you to have the freedom to make your own choices, so you're not relying on me to give you food plans for the rest of your life. Therefore, putting you on a diet as those, as we've discussed a thousand times, will never work!

To give you some suggestions to get you started, you will find some beautiful and detailed food plans and menu plans for all different ethnicities or eating preferences -vegans, vegetarians, meat eaters, pescatarians and even a no-cook plan. Also, the 5 food plans come with 58 delicious recipes that are amazing to try. Many of my clients say that these recipes quickly become firm favourites for all the family and continue to be so for many years.

Over the next few pages, you will find the different meal plans, including:

- General Food Plan
- 'No need to cook' Food Plan
- Vegan/Vegetarian Food Plan
- Pescatarian Food Plan
- Fruit Dinner Food Plan.

You will find the full recipes within each of these food plans and the Glycaemic Index Chart of high (and some low) blood sugar foods in your additional resources.

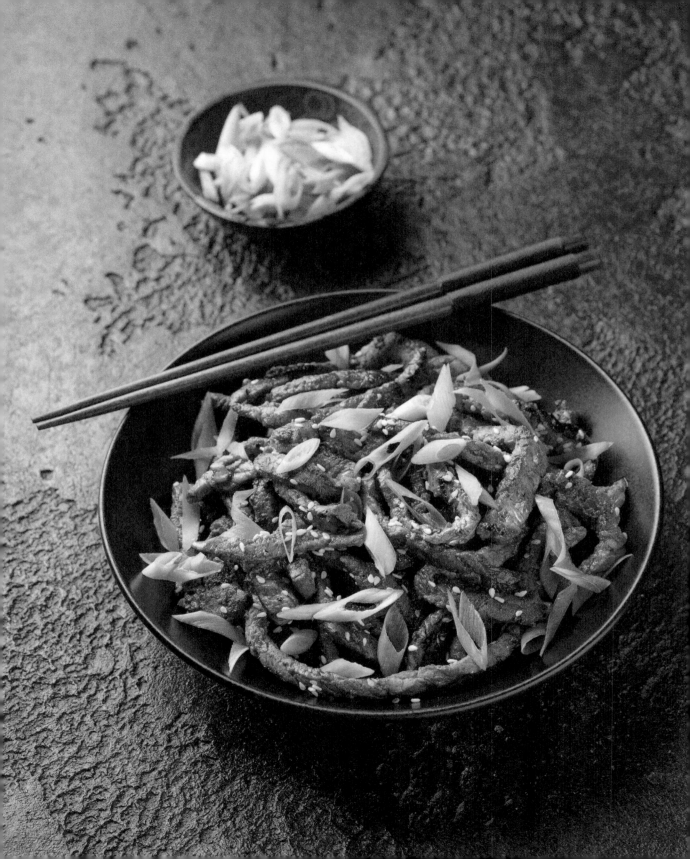

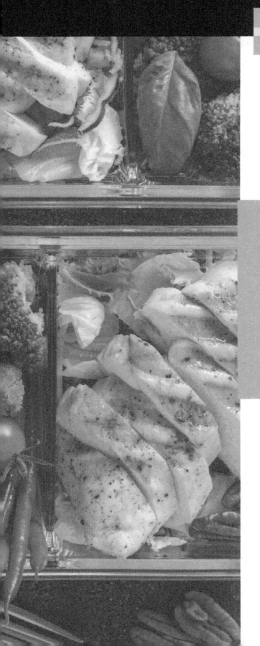

THE WEIGHT LOSS GURU

GENERAL
FOOD PLAN

CONTENTS

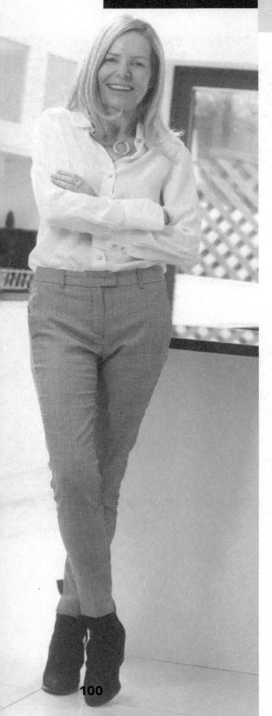

FOOD PLAN

FOOD PLAN

WEEK 1

	MON	TUE	WED	THUR	FRI	SAT	SUN
B'FAST	1 pot of Greek Yogurt & 1 Plant-based yogurt mixed together, (Fage+Alpro) + 2 tsp mixed seeds/nuts	2 eggs, scrambled with smoked salmon	Avocado with mushrooms	1 pot of Greek Yogurt & 1 Plant-based yogurt mixed together, (Fage+Alpro) + 2 tsp mixed seeds/nuts	2 kippers or haddock or mackerel	1 pot of Greek Yogurt & 1 Plant-based yogurt mixed together, (Fage+Alpro) + 2 tsp mixed seeds/nuts	Chia pot with almond milk, yogurt and prunes
LUNCH	Large serving of 'Oriental Chicken salad' + edamame beans	One large serving 'Lentil Pumpkin and Rocket Salad'	'Veal with Mustard Butter & Asparagus' + vegetables + butter beans	A large serving of 'Classic Niçoise Salad' + puy lentils	A large portion of 'Pancetta, Spinach & Ricotta Bake' + mixed vegetables	'Almond Lemon Cod' with spinach + lentils	A large portion of roast beef & courgettes with horseradish sauce + butter beans
TEA SNACK	2 pieces of fresh, seasonal fruit	2 pieces of fresh, seasonal fruit	2 pieces of fresh, seasonal fruit	2 pieces of fresh, seasonal fruit	2 pieces of fresh, seasonal fruit	2 pieces of fresh, seasonal fruit	2 pieces of fresh, seasonal fruit
SUPPER	'Thai Beef Salad' + small serving of hummus	A small serving of lamb chops + cannellini beans	A portion of 'Salmon Fillet with Spring Onions & soy sauce' + small serving of lentils	Three 'Scallops and Thai Pea Puree' + a small serving of lentils	'Salmon Fillet with Tiger Prawns' + a small serving of lentils	'Stuffed Marrow Bake' + a small serving of edamame beans	'Smoked Tofu Stir-Fry'

WEEK 2

	MON	TUE	WED	THUR	FRI	SAT	SUN
B'FAST	1 pot of Greek Yogurt & 1 Plant-based yogurt mixed together, (Fage+Alpro) + 2 tsp mixed seeds/nuts	Avocado with mushrooms	1 pot of Greek Yogurt & 1 Plant-based yogurt mixed together, (Fage+Alpro) + 2 tsp mixed seeds/nuts	2 kippers or haddock or mackerel	Chia pot with almond milk, yogurt and prunes	1 pot of Greek Yogurt & 1 Plant-based yogurt mixed together, (Fage+Alpro) + 2 tsp mixed seeds/nuts	2 eggs, scrambled with smoked salmon
LUNCH	Large portion of 'Mushroom & Fennel Salad' + edamame beans	A large portion of Butter bean and mushroom casserole with mixed vegetables	A large serving of 'Classic Niçoise Salad' + puy lentils	A large portion of 'Oriental Chicken Salad' + edamame beans	'Pesto-Crusted Cod' with a small serving of lentils	A large portion of 'Thai Beef Salad' + mixed vegetables	A large portion of roast chicken & mixed vegetables + pulse with gravy
TEA SNACK	2 pieces of fresh, seasonal fruit	2 pieces of fresh, seasonal fruit	2 pieces of fresh, seasonal fruit	2 pieces of fresh, seasonal fruit	2 pieces of fresh, seasonal fruit	2 pieces of fresh, seasonal fruit	2 pieces of fresh, seasonal fruit
SUPPER	Three 'Scallops and Thai Pea Puree' + a small serving of lentils	'Leek & Goats Cheese Frittata'	One pork steak + butter beans	'Split Pea, Green Peas Smoked Ham Soup'	'Lamb Kebabs' with a small portion of cannellini beans	Chicken soup + fava beans	'Devilled Tofu Kebabs'

101

*ALL RECIPES CAN BE FOUND IN YOUR ADDITIONAL RESOURCES

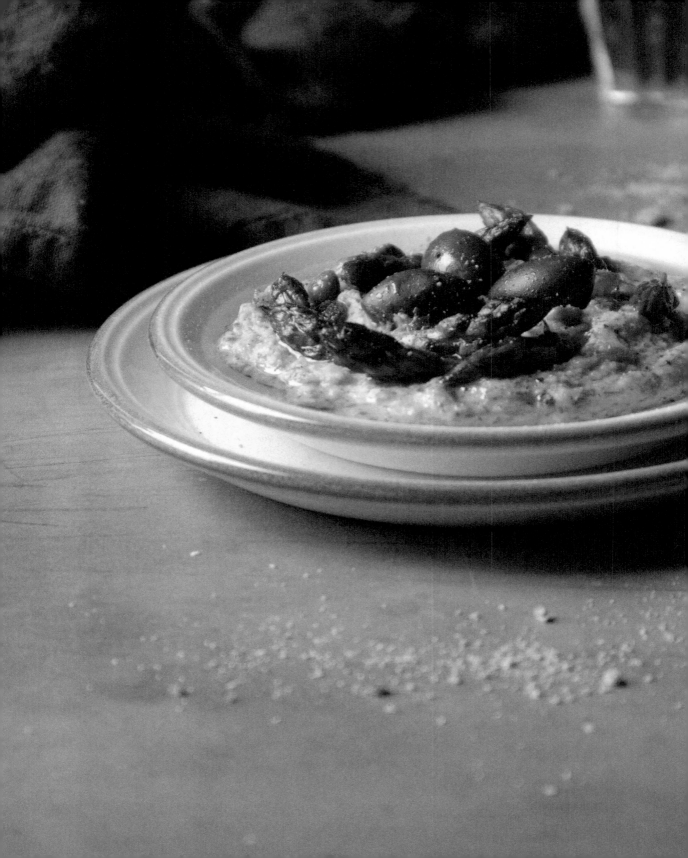

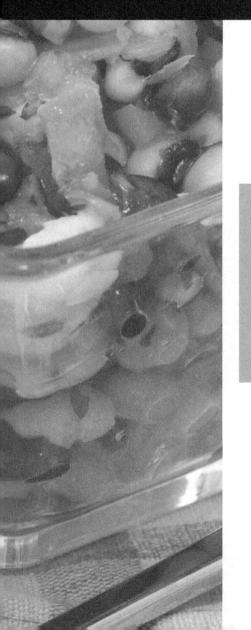

THE WEIGHT LOSS GURU

'NO NEED TO COOK'
FOOD PLAN

'NO NEED TO COOK' FOOD PLAN

	MON	TUE	WED	THUR	FRI	SAT	SUN
B'FAST	1 pot of Greek Yogurt & 1 Plant-based yogurt mixed together, (Fage+Alpro) + 2 tsp mixed seeds/nuts	Chia pot with almond milk, yogurt and prunes	½ avocado + cottage cheese	1 pot of Greek Yogurt & 1 Plant-based yogurt mixed together, (Fage+Alpro) + 2 tsp mixed seeds/nuts	2-3 kippers or haddock or mackerel	Chia pot with almond milk, yogurt and prunes	1 pot of Greek Yogurt & 1 Plant-based yogurt mixed together, (Fage+Alpro) + 2 tsp mixed seeds/nuts
LUNCH large portions	½ sachet Fiid of Chala Masala, ready cooked chicken + vegetables	½ sachet of Fiid, a packet of basil-flavoured tofu and Sainsbury's ready vegetables	Roasted tomato, cauliflower, pepper & tuna bake + cannellini beans	Pan baked gourmet lentils with fresh cherry tomatoes & feta + vegetables	Smoked mackerel fillets with Sainsbury's ready vegetables & Merchant lentils	Sainsbury's vegetable medley with baked cod + cannellini beans + large garden salad	M&S ready bought cauliflower, calamari, cherry tomatoes, 3-bean salad + feta
TEA SNACK	2 pieces of fresh, seasonal fruit	2 pieces of fresh, seasonal fruit	2 pieces of fresh, seasonal fruit	2 pieces of fresh, seasonal fruit	2 pieces of fresh, seasonal fruit	2 pieces of fresh, seasonal fruit	2 pieces of fresh, seasonal fruit
SUPPER	A whole packet of Sweet chilli Tiba brand tempeh	Quorn mince + small serving of kidney beans	Cauldron brand marinated tofu (microwave), add edamame & soy sauce	Smoked salmon & scrambled eggs	One packet of The Grocer brand - Red Lentil Dhal	A whole packet Curried flavour Tiba brand tempeh	Avocado and soy sauce filled with baked lentils and flaked salmon

WEEK 1

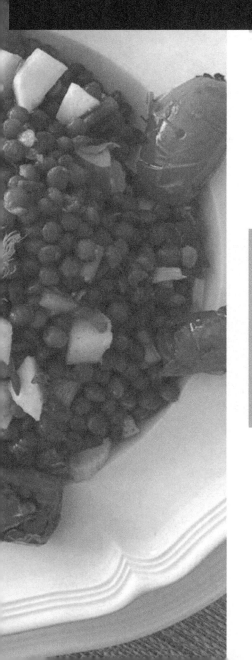

THE WEIGHT LOSS GURU

VEGAN/VEGETARIAN FOOD PLAN

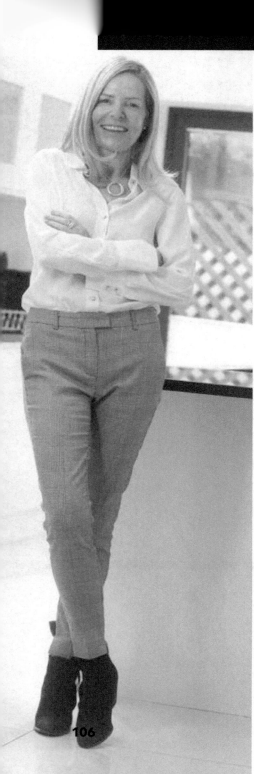

VEGAN / VEGETARIAN

1. SOFT TOFU SCRAMBLE
2. FALAFEL SALAD WITH HUMMUS
3. LENTIL, ROAST PUMPKIN & ROCKET SALAD
4. CAULIFLOWER & SPINACH CURRY
5. KALE SALAD
6. DEVILLED TOFU KEBABS
7. TECHNICOLOUR BEAN SALAD
8. TOFU, GREENS & CASHEW STIR-FRY
9. ROAST PUMPKIN & BROCCOLI SALAD
10. GREEN BEANS WITH RED ONION CONFIT
11. PUY LENTIL SALAD
12. CHICKPEA FRITTERS & TIKKA SAUCE
13. QUORN STUFFED MARROW BAKE
14. BUTTERBEAN & MUSHROOM CASSEROLE
15. SQUASH & CABBAGE SABZI
16. SMOKED TOFU & PEANUT STIR-FRY
17. SIMPLE VEGETABLE CURRY
18. EASY CAULIFLOWER DHAL
19. EGYPTIAN CALIFORNIA GARDEN
20. COURGETTE, PEA & PESTO SOUP
21. MUSHROOM & FENNEL SALAD
22. VEGGIE GOULASH
23. GINGER SWEET TOFU WITH PAK CHOI
24. BLACK-EYED BEAN MOLE WITH SALSA
25. TOFU ESCALOPES WITH BLACK OLIVE SALSA VERDE

VEGAN/VEGETARIAN FOOD PLAN

WEEK 1

	MON	TUE	WED	THUR	FRI	SAT	SUN
B'FAST	1 pot of vegan Greek Yogurt & 1 Plant-based yogurt mixed together + 2 tsp mixed seeds/nuts	Avocado & mushrooms	Chia pot with almond milk, yogurt and prunes	1 pot of vegan Greek Yogurt & 1 Plant-based yogurt mixed together + 2 tsp mixed seeds/nuts	Chia pot with almond milk, yogurt and prunes	Scrambled soft tofu	Grilled tomatoes, mushrooms and vegan bacon
LUNCH	A large portion of 'Falafel Salad with Hummus'	Large portion of 'Lentil, Pumpkin and Rocket Salad' + edamame beans	'Cauliflower & Spinach Curry' + large portion of lentils	A large portion of 'Kale Salad' + vegetables & cannellini beans	A large serving of 'Black-Eyed Bean Mole with Salsa' + broccoli and sauerkraut	'Devilled Tofu Kebabs' + steamed vegetables & hummus	One serving of 'Tofu Escalopes with Black Olive Salsa Verde' + lentils
TEA SNACK	2 pieces of fresh, seasonal fruit	2 pieces of fresh, seasonal fruit	2 pieces of fresh, seasonal fruit	2 pieces of fresh, seasonal fruit	2 pieces of fresh, seasonal fruit	2 pieces of fresh, seasonal fruit	2 pieces of fresh, seasonal fruit
SUPPER	'Veggie Goulash with Quorn or Tofu'	'Technicolour Bean Salad'	'Smoked Tofu Kebabs'	'Tofu & Cashew Stir-Fry'	'Roast Pumpkin & Broccoli Salad'	Large portion of Tarka dahl	'Green Beans with Red Onion Confit' + small portion of cannellini beans

WEEK 2

	MON	TUE	WED	THUR	FRI	SAT	SUN
B'FAST	1 pot of vegan Greek Yogurt & 1 Plant-based yogurt mixed together + 2 tsp mixed seeds/nuts	Chia pot with almond milk, yogurt and prunes	Avocado & mushrooms	1 pot of vegan Greek Yogurt & 1 Plant-based yogurt mixed together + 2 tsp mixed seeds/nuts	Chia pot with almond milk, yogurt and prunes	Scrambled soft tofu	Grilled tomatoes, mushrooms and vegan bacon
LUNCH	A large portion of 'Puy Lentil Salad' + steamed vegetables	Large serving of 'Mushroom & Fennel Salad' + hummus	'Chickpea Fritters & Tikka Sauce' + broccoli and cannellini beans	A large portion of 'Quorn Stuffed Marrow Bake' + large garden salad + lentils	'Butterbean & Mushroom Casserole' + vegetables + sauerkraut	A large serving of ' Squash & Cabbage Sabzi' + large garden salad + hummus	'Smoked Tofu & Peanut Stir-Fry' + steamed vegetables and hummus
TEA SNACK	2 pieces of fresh, seasonal fruit	2 pieces of fresh, seasonal fruit	2 pieces of fresh, seasonal fruit	2 pieces of fresh, seasonal fruit	2 pieces of fresh, seasonal fruit	2 pieces of fresh, seasonal fruit	2 pieces of fresh, seasonal fruit
SUPPER	'Simple Vegetable Curry'	'Easy Cauliflower Dahl'	'Ginger Sweet Tofu & Pak Choi'	'California Garden'	'Smoked Tofu Kebabs'	Chilli Con Carne with Quorn mince	'Courgette, Pea & Pesto Soup' + a small portion of lentils

*ALL RECIPES CAN BE FOUND IN YOUR ADDITIONAL RESOURCES

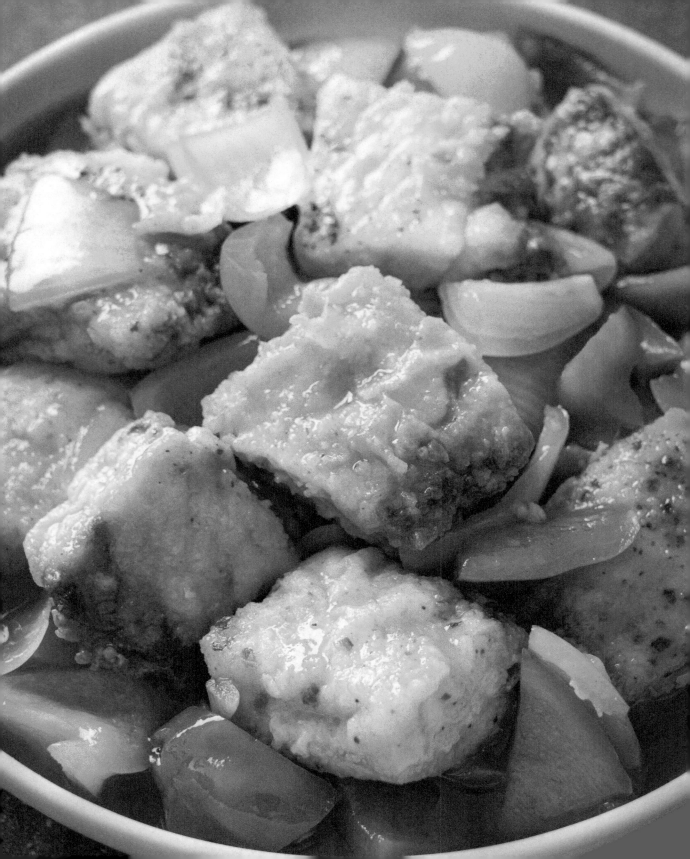

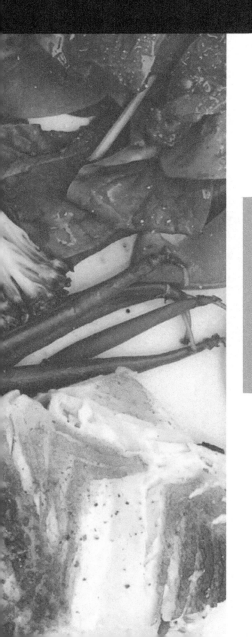

THE WEIGHT LOSS GURU

PESCATARIAN FOOD PLAN

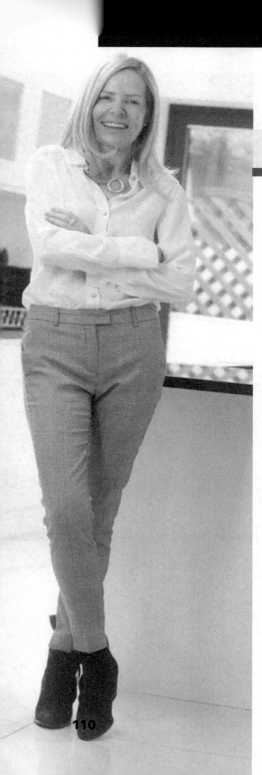

PESCATARIAN FOOD PLAN

1. ALMOND LEMON COD
2. BUTTER BEAN AND MUSHROOM CASSEROLE
3. CHILLI GARLIC PRAWNS
4. COURGETTE, PEA & PESTO SOUP
5. GRILLED GOATS CHEESE ON MUSHROOM
6. LEEK & GOATS CHEESE FRITTATA
7. LENTIL, ROAST PUMPKIN, FETA & ROCKET SALAD
8. PESTO-CRUSTED COD WITH PUY LENTILS
9. PARMESAN FRITTATA
10. CLASSIC SALAD NICOISE
11. SALMON FILLET WITH TIGER PRAWNS
12. SALMON WITH SPRING ONIONS AND SOY SAUCE
13. SCALLOPS WITH THAI-SCENTED PEA PUREE
14. SOFT TOFU SCRAMBLE
15. STUFFED MARROW BAKE
16. PUY LENTIL & HALLOUMI SALAD
17. SMOKED TOFU & PEANUT STIR-FRY
18. DEVILLED TOFU KEBABS
19. TOFU, GREENS & CASHEW STIR-FRY
20. ORIENTAL VEGAN CHICKEN SALAD
21. FALAFEL SALAD WITH HUMMUS
22. ROAST PUMPKIN, BROCCOLI SALAD

PESCATARIAN FOOD PLAN

	MON	TUE	WED	THUR	FRI	SAT	SUN
B'FAST	1 pot of Greek Yogurt & 1 Plant-based yogurt mixed together, (Fage+Alpro) + 2 tsp mixed seeds/nuts	Chia pot with almond milk, yogurt and prunes	1 pot of Greek Yogurt & 1 Plant-based yogurt mixed together, (Fage+Alpro) + 2 tsp mixed seeds/nuts	Poached egg & sliced smoked salmon	1 pot of Greek Yogurt & 1 Plant-based yogurt mixed together, (Fage+Alpro) + 2 tsp mixed seeds/nuts	2 kippers or haddock or mackerel	Chia pot with almond milk, yogurt and prunes
LUNCH	A portion of 'Salmon Fillet & Tiger Prawns' + puy lentils + vegetables	One large serving of 'Classic Salad Nicoise' + edamame beans	A large serving of 'Pesto-Crusted Cod + Puy Lentils' + vegetables	Large 'Scallops & Thai-Scented Pea Puree' + steamed vegetables + edamame beans	'Devilled Tofu Kebabs' + sauerkraut + a portion of vegetables	A portion of Salmon Fillet & Tiger Prawns' + puy lentils + vegetables	'Almond Lemon Cod' + large garden salad and puy lentils
TEA SNACK	2 portions of fresh, seasonal fruit	2 portions of fresh, seasonal fruit	2 portions of fresh, seasonal fruit	2 portions of fresh, seasonal fruit	2 portions of fresh, seasonal fruit	2 portions of fresh, seasonal fruit	2 portions of fresh, seasonal fruit
SUPPER	'Chilli Garlic Prawns' + small portion of lentils	'Almond Lemon Cod' + small serving of puy lentils	'Soft Tofu Scramble' +	'Chilli Garlic Prawns' + small portion of edamame beans	A portion of 'Salmon Fillet with Spring Onions & soy sauce' + small serving of lentils	A large portion of 'Tarka dal'	One portion of 'Classic Salad Nicoise'

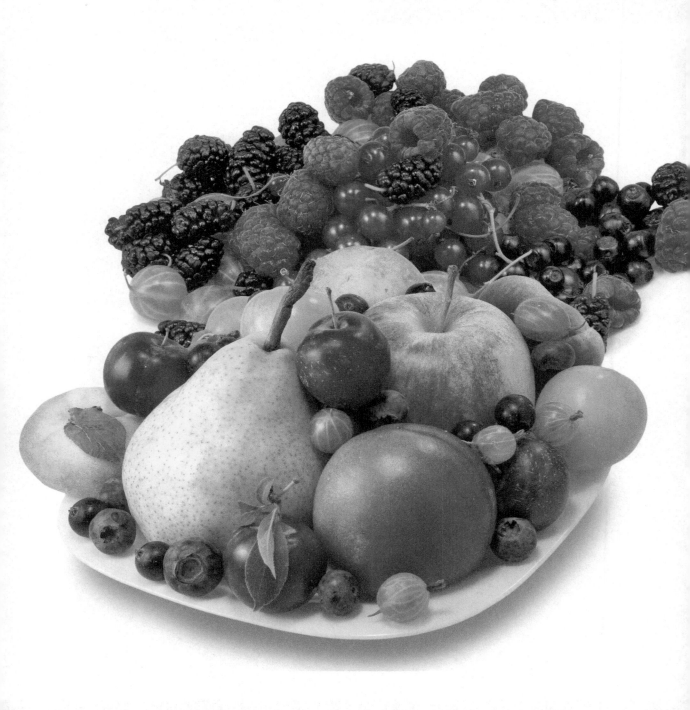

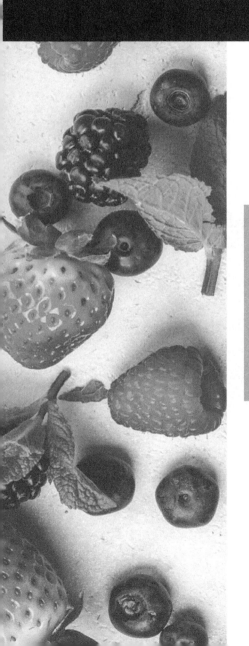

THE WEIGHT LOSS GURU

FRUIT DINNER
FOOD PLAN

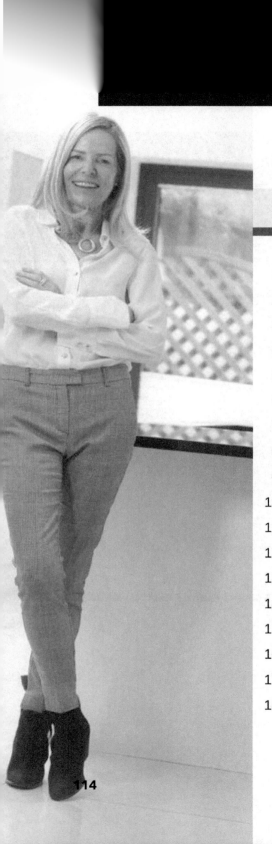

FRUIT DINNER FOOD PLAN

1. ORIENTAL CHICKEN SALAD
2. LENTIL, ROAST PUMPKIN, FETA & ROCKET SALAD
3. CLASSIC SALAD NICOISE
4. CRISPY PANCETTA, SPINACH & RICOTTA BAKE
5. SALMON WITH SPRING ONIONS & SOY SAUCE
6. SALMON FILLET WITH TIGER PRAWNS
7. STUFFED MARROW BAKE
8. SMOKED TOFU & PEANUT STIR-FRY
9. SPLIT PEA & GREEN PEA SMOKED HAM SOUP
10. THAI BEEF SALAD
11. SCALLOPS WITH THAI-SCENTED PEA PUREE
12. LEEK GOATS CHEESE FRITTATA
13. BUTTER BEAN AND MUSHROOM CASSEROLE
14. PESTO-CRUSTED COD WITH PUY LENTILS
15. CHILLI GARLIC PRAWNS
16. COURGETTE, PEA & PESTO SOUP
17. SALMON, ASPARAGUS & PEA SALAD
18. MUSHROOM SALAD

FRUIT DINNER FOOD PLAN

WEEK 1

	MON	TUE	WED	THUR	FRI	SAT	SUN
B'FAST	1 pot of Greek Yogurt & 1 Plant-based yogurt mixed together, (Fage+Alpro) + 2 tsp mixed seeds/nuts	2 eggs, scrambled with smoked salmon	Chia pot with almond milk, yogurt and prunes	1 pot of Greek Yogurt & 1 Plant-based yogurt mixed together, (Fage+Alpro) + 2 tsp mixed seeds/nuts	2 kippers or haddock or mackerel	1 pot of Greek Yogurt & 1 Plant-based yogurt mixed together, (Fage+Alpro) + 2 tsp mixed seeds/nuts	Mushroom Omelette
LUNCH	Large serving of 'Oriental Chicken Salad' + edamame beans	Large serving of 'Lentil, Pumpkin & Rocket salad' + hummus + sauerkraut	Large serving of 'Salmon, Asparagus & Pea Salad' + lentils	Large serving of 'Classic Salad Niçoise' with green beans + puy lentils	A large portion of 'Pancetta, Spinach & Ricotta Bake' + salad	A serving of 'Pesto-Crusted Cod with Puy Lentils' + spinach	A large portion of roast beef & courgettes with horseradish sauce + butter beans
FRUIT GRAZE (3-6PM)	5 - 6 portions of fresh, seasonal fruit to be grazed on between 3 - 6pm	5 - 6 portions of fresh, seasonal fruit to be grazed on between 3 - 6pm	5 - 6 portions of fresh, seasonal fruit to be grazed on between 3 - 6pm	5 - 6 portions of fresh, seasonal fruit to be grazed on between 3 - 6pm	5 - 6 portions of fresh, seasonal fruit to be grazed on between 3 - 6pm	5 - 6 portions of fresh, seasonal fruit to be grazed on between 3 - 6pm	5 - 6 portions of fresh, seasonal fruit to be grazed on between 3 - 6pm

WEEK 2

	MON	TUE	WED	THUR	FRI	SAT	SUN
B'FAST	1 pot of Greek Yogurt & 1 Plant-based yogurt mixed together, (Fage+Alpro) + 2 tsp mixed seeds/nuts	Avocado and mushrooms	1 pot of Greek Yogurt & 1 Plant-based yogurt mixed together, (Fage+Alpro) + 2 tsp mixed seeds/nuts	Chia pot with almond milk, yogurt and prunes	2 kippers or haddock or mackerel	1 pot of Greek Yogurt & 1 Plant-based yogurt mixed together, (Fage+Alpro) + 2 tsp mixed seeds/nuts	Mushroom Omelette
LUNCH	Large portion of 'Mushroom Salad' with fennel + edamame beans	A large serving of ' Courgette, Pea & Pesto Soup' + large garden salad + lentils	Large serving of 'Classic Salad Niçoise' with green beans + edamame beans	A large serving of 'Scallops with Thai-Scented Pea-Puree' + vegetables + lentils	A large serving of 'Split Pea, Green Pea & Smoked Ham soup + butter beans	A large serving of 'Thai Beef Salad' + butter beans	A large portion of roast chicken & mixed vegetables + pulse with gravy
FRUIT GRAZE (3-6PM)	5 - 6 portions of fresh fruit to be grazed on between 3 - 6pm	5 - 6 portions of fresh fruit to be grazed on between 3 - 6pm	5 - 6 portions of fresh fruit to be grazed on between 3 - 6pm	5 - 6 portions of fresh fruit to be grazed on between 3 - 6pm	5 - 6 portions of fresh fruit to be grazed on between 3 - 6pm	5 - 6 portions of fresh fruit to be grazed on between 3 - 6pm	5 - 6 portions of fresh fruit to be grazed on between 3 - 6pm

*ALL RECIPES CAN BE FOUND IN YOUR ADDITIONAL RESOURCES

Breakfast List

Eggs, smoked salmon, plain omelette, avocado, mushroom omelette, kippers, haddock, Greek yoghurt, protein yoghurt, mushrooms, chicken, mung bean porridge, chia pot with almond milk, scrambled tofu, Turkey bacon.

Please treat these as a starting place and not a prescription. If you don't like something or it doesn't work for your lifestyle, swap it for something else. For example, if you love a meal and want to have it every day, go ahead! Work with the principles in chapter 3 and make plans of your own.

Troubleshooting

When I work directly with a client, we can fine-tune things. What works for one person might not work for another. Things change as you lose fat and your insulin resistance and metabolism start to recover. If you lose a lot of weight, your BMR could also shift dramatically.

The tips in this section are suggestions for things you might like to experiment with if you struggle to lose weight at first or hit a plateau later. Read through them and see if something resonates with you. If it does, then that might be the perfect place to start.

Portion Sizes

It's not healthy to weigh or measure your food as it smacks at an eating disorder. This is all normal eating. The way it should always have been. It would help if you didn't feel restricted. If you are hungry, then you should eat! As your body starts to recover and work well, you will find that you can eat a phenomenal amount of the right foods. Once you are insulin sensitive rather than insulin resistant, your body starts to talk to you. Also, eating less of those insulin-inducing starches means you'll find that when you're eating right, you will feel full. Those starches (processed sugars) were making you hungry all the time.

The important thing is to listen to your body. Are you genuinely hungry or just thirsty? Or bored? How much do you need to eat to feel satisfied? Aim to eat until you are no longer hungry rather than stuffed. It's perfectly fine to stop before you finish everything on your plate (no matter what your parents told you when you were little!) You can find out more about this in chapter 8.

For breakfast, think large restaurant-sized portion. You want to eat as much as they would serve you in a quality restaurant and a little more. That's why the double pot of yoghurts with seeds and nuts works so well.

For lunch, think pub grub size – a more significant portion size than a typical restaurant. Don't forget lunch – as it used to be for many centuries previously – is the main meal of the day. Food is energy. Food is your daytime medicine. So have a large lunch and enjoy it. If you like measuring at lunchtime, think about three palms worth of pulses and vegetables and two palms of protein.

Fruit is your afternoon snack, so if just a snack (not a fruit dinner), then one or two pieces, such as a satsuma and an apple in winter and some strawberries and raspberries in summer. Dinner is your smallest meal. From 6pm onwards, how much will you generally be moving on most evenings? For dinner, imagine a plate in a posh restaurant. That's usually about the right portion size. It fills just the middle of the plate. That might be a protein portion the size of the palm of your hand and the same or a bit less for your pulse.

Two times per week guide

As I say elsewhere, there are a few anomalies, so I like to give a little guide here. Salmon, avocado, cottage cheese, prawns, humus and eggs are very high in calories, fat, or both. So, the simplest way to think is don't restrict yourself but with those foods, let's always say a maximum of twice a week. That's easy to do and gives you a balanced way of eating.

SALE – sugar, alcohol, late eating

For 99% of my clients, the way to have guaranteed success is to focus on these three things. Get these right, and you're well on the way to a permanent healthy lifestyle of weight loss and easy maintenance.

Sugar – examples are – bread, pasta, rice, potatoes, cakes, biscuits, crisps, and chocolate. These are processed artificial starches (you never eat uncooked rice or potato from the ground unprocessed!), and these foods are for bulking. So, if you are a full-on athlete, child, labourer, farmer, hunter or gatherer, then go for it. For anyone else, these are almost the sole reason you aren't your dream weight. Swap these out with pulses during the weight management stage, and the results will be outstanding.

Alcohol - (read the chapter on alcohol), but when you remember that every single unit you have is the equivalent of one chocolate bar, then very simply, the more you reduce your intake (during this weight management stage), the quicker and more successful the results you'll get.

Late eating – (read the chapter on Eating Times), but if you count backwards 4 hours before bed, you eat your dinner as many nights as you can at this time. Then, every night you do this, you will lose weight, as for the first time in many years, you'll eat rather than store fat!

Fat

Fat is very high in energy. We know that for every gram of fat there are 9 calories. Therefore, if you eat more energy than you need, it will be stored as fat in your body, so most of us need to be careful not to overeat with these high-energy foods.

Fats are essential to your diet - if you eat the right ones. Lots of lovely foods like nuts, seeds, avocado, fish and olives are full of healthy fats, and you certainly do not have to avoid them! Please include them in your meals, sprinkle them on salads, and have oily fish a few times a week (unless you are vegetarian or vegan). Remember that you don't have to add extra fat to your plate - it's already in the food.

Cheese

We need to talk about one type of fat a bit more - cheese.

Cheese is a very high-fat food (generally, the harder the cheese, the higher its fat content will be). Unfortunately, it's also so moreish that it's almost addictive. Very often, a new client will tell me that they don't eat much cheese, but when I dig a little deeper, it's in almost every meal or has a habit of sneaking in.

Considering every slice of cheese is 300 calories, and your BMR might be 1200 calories, then if you have 4 slices of cheese in one day, that is your whole calorie allowance for the entire day! After that, you wouldn't be able to eat another thing, let alone crackers and butter!

Not only that, but cheese also has really no nutritional value. It causes asthma and eczema, makes your breath smell and is terrible for your skin. So, if you had never tasted cheese and were presented with the facts, it's unlikely you would choose to eat it.

I'm not going to tell you to give up cheese if you don't want to. So go and enjoy some feta on a salad or grate a little cheddar on a vegetable bake. Just be aware of how much you're having. Indeed, don't sit and nibble on slices of cheese as a snack without realising how much you've eaten.

Again, with cottage cheese, I find some new clients start to dollop it on everything. This is something to be avoided. Adding this creamy, fatty food slows weight loss, so have it only twice a week.

Nuts

Nuts and seeds contain lovely nutrients and can be very good for you. I recommend sprinkling seeds on your breakfast, and it's OK to include walnuts in a salad or make a peanut sauce. In the weight loss phase, it is essential to be aware that nuts are high in fat. While this is good fat and not something you have to avoid, it does mean that a packet of nuts could easily contain 600 calories – a third of the energy you need for the day. You could have a satisfying meal with the same number of calories.

If you snack on nuts, especially if you eat while distracted by the TV or even at work, it's easy to consume that whole packet without noticing. Of course, many flavoured or roasted nuts also have added sugar, which we want to avoid. The best approach is to include nuts and seeds in meals but never snack on them.

Snacks and Fruit

The best food for a snack is always fruit. All those protein bars, protein balls, *Deliciously Ella* snacks, *Kind, Tribe, and Renegade* bars are just sugar by another name. They are made of nuts, and dried fruit - particularly dates (GI 105) and honey (GI 87). They might be a bit healthier than a *Snickers* or a *Twix,* but not really. Animals - humans- are supposed to have six teaspoons of natural sugar per day from natural carbs - fruit, veg, salad, spice, seeds and pulses. Why would anyone need these processed sugar insulin-induced snacks, unless in training or a manual job?

So, when it comes to snacks, it's best to stick with fruit. You also want to avoid high GI fruits such as watermelon, pineapple, melon, banana, kiwi, mango, and dried fruits like dates and raisins. Exotic fruits like those contain a lot of fast-acting sugar and can be very high GI, even higher than white sugar! They grow in different climates and are tailored to animals with additional needs. You are not a monkey; you don't need to eat bananas.

It's also important to always eat your fruit raw and on its own. Studies have shown that just a handful of blueberries a day lowers blood pressure, but only when eaten on their own. Suppose you mix any berry with dairy - like blueberries and Greek yoghurt or strawberries and cream. In that case, the beneficial nutrients are blocked and don't get to your bloodstream.

Avocados are an excellent fruit, full of iron, copper, potassium, monosaturated fats, and vitamin E. Still, a whole avocado has somewhere between 200 – 300 calories. So during the weight management stage, maybe two per week is optimal.

Vegetables

There are so many delicious vegetables that you can use as the basis for your meals. From mushrooms, cabbage, aubergine, cauliflower, spinach and courgette, you can pile your plate high and enjoy!

However, there are two things to be aware of. First, some vegetables are full of faster-acting carbohydrates, also known as high GI foods, and are best avoided while losing weight. They include sweeter vegetables like sweetcorn and some root vegetables. Quickly look at a GI chart if you are struggling to shift fat. You want to aim to eat things that come in under 40.

Seafood

Generally, fish and seafood are excellent and healthy options. If they are high in fat, it's almost always the good kind. There are a few to be aware of, though. Lobster is relatively high in cholesterol; you'll know it is also very rich if you eat dark crab meat. As a salmon fillet can provide up to 275 calories, I

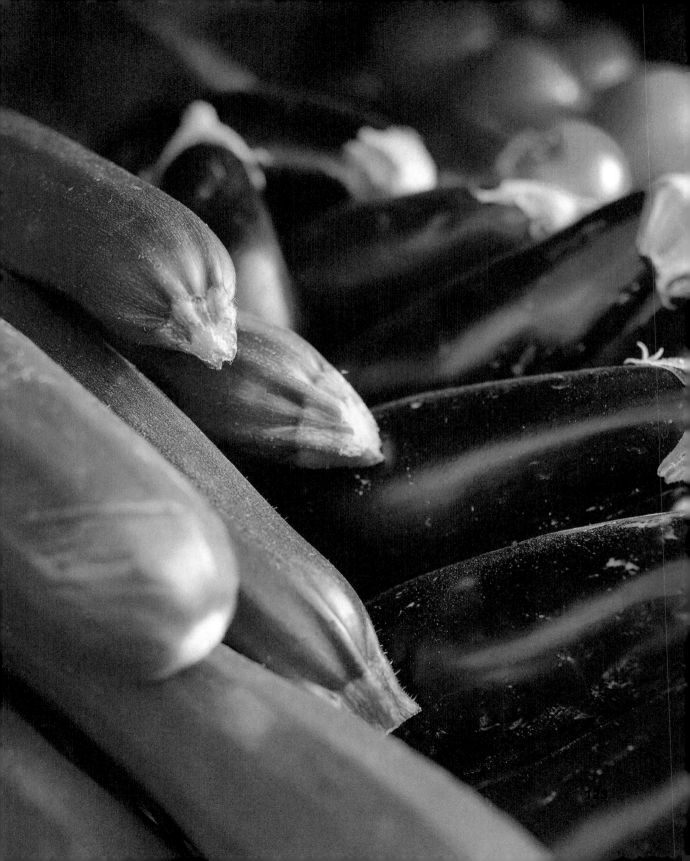

recommend salmon only twice weekly. Many of my clients at the beginning start adding salmon to most meals which means they are moving from sugars to fats – something to be avoided. These might be things to keep an eye on if you eat them regularly.

Prawns cause some of my client's problems as well. There's nothing wrong with prawns, but I have noticed that often when my clients eat them, they don't lose weight. People rarely cook prawns without frying them in butter or smothering them in a creamy sauce. All that added fat stalls your weight loss, but it's better to avoid temptation and give prawns a miss if they are problematic for you while you're in the weight loss phase. Of course, if you like your prawns plain, they are a great source of protein!

Couscous and Quinoa

Quinoa is a rice-pulse that has a GI of 54, which is just lower than white sugar. It is more a grain than a seed. Again, during the weight management stage, this is something I would avoid. Likewise, many people think couscous is a healthy food. Still, it is pasta with a GI of 64, equivalent to a croissant. I am not trying to demonise food here, but who needs food with a GI index equal to a croissant?!

Gluten-free Foods

People sometimes think that gluten-free food (like pasta or bread) will not have processed carbohydrates and will be a healthier choice. Unfortunately, this is rarely the case. A gluten-free diet is simply one that avoids wheat and a few other grains. Usually, manufacturers of gluten-free products replace wheat flour with rice flour, which might seem like a simple enough swap. But unfortunately, rice flour has a much higher GI than wheat flour. Not only that, but it also has almost no flavour, so there is likely to be a few spoonsful of sugar added to make it edible.

Whether you have a medical need to avoid gluten or not, it's usually best to cut out any wheat-based food rather than turn to alternatives.

Eating Out

I love eating out, and so do many of my clients. It's so easy to eat well in a good restaurant! Almost any fish dish will be a delicious and healthy option, which are my favourites. Still, any protein dish is a great choice. Refrain from ordering sugary sides like bread, pasta, potatoes or rice.

You may lose slightly less weight on the days you eat late at a restaurant, but that doesn't matter since not many people eat out every night. If you eat out three or four times a week, you could try having fruit for dinner (option three in chapter 5) on the other nights if you want to boost your weight loss, but that's up to you.

Eating when travelling with work.

Many of my clients struggle with their eating habits when travelling for work. Being away from your usual foods, shops and routines is discombobulating. So for some, it's almost as though being abroad means all the sense and simplicity of this healthy eating lifestyle goes out the window. Suddenly they have to go back to their old unhealthy ways or worse! So what I always suggest here is simple. The first night you arrive, have some fun. See some friends or colleagues, eat, drink, go to bed late; do whatever you want to do and feel that you've arrived.

Well done to you for achieving this work position and the level you represent your business abroad. Then, the very next morning, everything changes. Just imagine that you will be where you are now for the next two years, not two days or two weeks, the next two years. What would you do differently, then? First, you should start working out where the healthier supermarkets are, where there is somewhere for you to work out. Buy some weights for your hotel room. See if the hotel has a fitness area. Work out where you will get the best lunch choices if you are out at meetings all day. Spending time abroad or travelling with work doesn't mean you need to give up your healthy lifestyle and eating choices – far from it. You don't want to set yourself onto a roller coaster lifestyle of healthy when at home and bingeing when away. That's not going to help anybody!

Sleep

Sleep is essential in the weight loss journey. If you are tired, you will always want to grab something to give you energy - which often means sugar. An early dinner should mean that you are getting better sleep. Still, if something else is disturbing you, it might be worth seeing if there's anything you can do about it. For example, if drinking extra water during the day means getting up at night to go to the loo, you should aim to consume most of your water earlier in the day and have less from mid-afternoon onwards. Typically all my clients comment that once they stop eating dinner or snacks so late that it wakes them up when they should be going into rest mode, their sleep improves once they are on this program.

Stress

We know that high insulin levels lead to weight gain. If you eat lots of sugar, your blood sugar rises, you release insulin, and the blood glucose is stored as fat. Unfortunately, stress has the same effect. When stressed, your body produces adrenaline and goes into a fight or flight mode. Your blood sugar rises, preparing to fuel your muscles while you run or battle. If you don't do that exercise, you will release lots of insulin to deal with the high blood sugar, which means you store fat. As with sleep, if you are very stressed, it will make it harder to lose weight (and isn't good for you generally), so it may be worth seeing if there's anything you could do to reduce your stress level.

For some people, stress also leads to emotional eating. You can find out more about dealing with that in chapter 8.

Inflammation

Inflammation in the body can lead to insulin resistance. This can be because of inflammatory compounds that slow the way insulin works. This leads to higher glucose levels, and fat accumulation in the liver which can further exacerbate insulin resistance. They can then start to fuel one another, causing a vicious cycle: weight gain causes more insulin resistance, and insulin resistance leads to more weight gain. Inflammation might come from an injury or medical condition. It also rises when women become menopausal or peri-menopausal; the drop in oestrogen means joints are less well-protected than before. A natural anti-inflammatory like turmeric (with black pepper and ginger) may help. Having said that, you will still lose weight if you are filling up all day on proteins, carbohydrates (fruits, vegetables, seeds etc.), fats and avoiding sugars.

Constipation

One little word of note. Suppose you've been living for years on toxins like alcohol, cigarettes, coffee, and heavy breads. In that case, these could have been assisting you in emptying your bowels. Not necessarily in a healthy way, but as you know, nothing gets you rushing to the loo quicker than a gin and tonic, and cigarette. Once you start eating healthily on this plan, you'll find that you're going to the loo more often as you're eating more good carbs and pulses.

But if you suffer constipation during the transition, going from a heavy toxin eater to a healthy eater, here are a few solutions I offer all clients ranging from stage 1 to stage 2 and finally stage 3.

Stage 1

Some women's bowels change after childbirth and find they are a little constipated to start with if eating fewer bulking agents like bread or cereal than they used to. In this case, I recommend putting two teaspoons of that lovely oatmeal (not oats) into your yoghurt, seed, and nut mix every morning. Oatmeal is so fine that it doesn't store fat down into the bowels, unlike certain sugary cereals. But it just sits at the bottom of the bowel, filling that space as the oatmeal expands whilst it sits there.

As I mentioned before, I lived in Asia for 7 years. I learnt from the best that many of those Chinese teas are being served all over Asia and are very cleverly designed to speed up digestion and aid regular body cleansing. Some are too much, so take care. Living in Thailand, for example, taught me there is tremendous pressure to be extremely thin – not in a healthy way. Many girls use these teas almost as a laxative, so be careful. However, these innocent teas here that I show are nature's way which is primarily fennel and artichoke. They are nature's way of being regular and no harm in having one per day if feeling a bit blocked up.

Stage 2

Suppose the above has yet to work, and you are still slightly struggling. In that case, I recommend purchasing and consuming papaya enzyme or fresh papaya until your bowels return to their normal state. Papaya is also nature's way of ensuring regulated bowel emptying. However, a little is more extreme than the fennel or artichoke options. We should do number two every single day of our lives for the best health. Finding fresh papaya around all year round is only sometimes achievable, so those lovely people at Holland & Barret have done the job for you and extracted the essence that you need to achieve results.

Stage 3

This is the only way I recommend that it is unnatural, so be careful with quantities. You want to avoid finding yourself using these as a laxative regularly. Laxatee and Slimatee can be bought over the counter in any chemist or pharmacy. Still, they do contain senna, so use them with precaution.

All the above suggestions help but rest assured, eventually, you will attend to number two more regularly. This plan can provide life-changing improvements for many clients suffering from Hashimoto, Crohn's disease and IBS.

Yasmin, David and Sophie

Yasmin

Yasmin has had yoghurt and fruit for breakfast, which she always thought was a healthy option. She had seen articles calling berries "superfoods" and was quite proud of herself for eating a handful daily. However, now she knows that the yoghurt was stopping them from being absorbed properly, she will have yoghurt, nuts and seeds for breakfast and save her berries for a morning snack.

David

David used to live on ready meals and takeaways, so planning his own meals was a challenge. He has undoubtedly been using ready-cooked products, especially pulses. Still, he's never entirely sure how to combine them into meals. However, having looked at the No-Cook Meal Plan, David feels much more confident.

He will follow the meal plan for a week to get a feel for it and try out some new foods, then he'll take his favourite meals and add them to the ones he is already eating.

Sophie

Although Sophie now eats dinner with her children, she has been making separate meals, something more traditional for them and a high-protein dish for herself. After reading this chapter, she sees that she has been doing more work than she needed to! Dinner time will be much easier now that she will be eating the same foods she cooks for the rest of the family, just cutting out the junk.

Where the children have the starches such as pasta and rice, she will replace them with a pulse such as butter beans or chickpeas. She will have mince and kidney beans whereas they have mince and pasta. She will have chicken and butter beans when they have chicken and roast potatoes. It's so simple she now sees!

Over to You

Did anything jump out at you as you read through this chapter? You may have been inspired by new meal ideas, or maybe there's something that you want to tweak. Now is the time to journal your thoughts and plan to implement them in the next week.

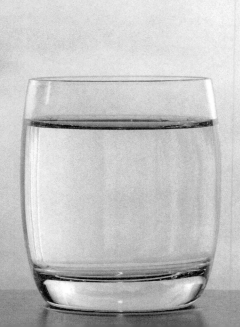

L - Liquids for Life

"According to experts, water is ranked second only to oxygen as essential for life. With more than half of your body weight made of water, you couldn't survive for more than a few days without it. On the other hand, you can survive without food for weeks."
- College of Tropical Agriculture and
Human Resources University of Hawaii at Manoa

We are almost halfway through the seven simple steps and have looked at **R**eal food, **E**ating times and **C**utting the junk. Next in the **RECLAIM** acronym is **L**, which stands for **L**iquids. We will be addressing alcohol in detail in the next chapter. For now, I'll focus on the many other liquids that we all consume, often daily. Starting with the most important one - water.

Water

Water is essential for all of us. In fact, we are living sponges, and dehydration contributes to many health issues. When you hear that your brain is 73% water, it's not surprising that dehydration can easily lead to migraines and headaches! Blood has an even higher water content at 92%, so it's clear that water is vital for good health. In fact, cabin crew, who spend their whole working lives in the dry atmosphere of an aeroplane, can have organs 10 years older than they should be. This is because they age 10 years due to dehydration.

These are just some of the things that water does for you:

- Carries nutrients and oxygen to your cells
- Suppresses your appetite
- Helps your digestive system work well
- Normalises your blood pressure
- Helps regulate your body temperature
- Stimulates your metabolism
- Lubricates your joints
- Flushes bacteria from your bladder
- Makes exercise more effective
- Helps metabolise fat
- Maintains proper electrolyte (sodium) balance
- Protects your tissues and organs
- Reduces stress

Ideally, you want your body to be 60% water, but often it's much lower. When some of my clients first step on a smart scale, their body water measurement might be as low as 30%, which means they are 70% "dry weight". When you talk about weight loss, you are only ever talking about dry weight. You never want to lose wet weight, so if you are 60% water, your dry weight is only 40%, making it considerably easier to lose that fat.

To stay hydrated and get all these benefits for weight loss and health, you should drink around 3 litres of water per day. But, of course, we only want to be measuring and calculating some of the time, so one approach, which

I love, is to drink a glass of water for every hour you're awake. It's so simple! Just one glass of water every hour, and you could quickly drink 15 or 16 glasses daily and hit that 3-litre target with little effort. This approach keeps you hydrated throughout the day, and you are never faced with the prospect of drinking 2l at 8 pm. But, of course, if you manage to do it, it will inevitably mean getting up at night! Alternatively, buy a large water jug from Amazon. Have it by your side all day to remind you and ensure you have finished it by 8 pm latest in the day.

Think about it, what time did you wake up this morning? How long have you been awake, and have you had that many glasses of water? Probably not! Most people live with a low level of dehydration every day. It affects many things, not just headaches but also your kidney and liver function, skin and even hair. In addition, humans often can't tell the difference between hunger and thirst, so if you constantly feel peckish, you might need more water.

Water retention makes you bloated.

Ironically, water retention is often caused by drinking too little water. Suppose you have a bloated belly or even NAFLD (non-alcoholic fatty liver disease). In that case, it might be caused by your drinking too little water. A camel's hump is not made of water. It is made of fat. Camels can live without water or food for around 10 days. They are adapted to the desert condition to an extent where they store lots of energy in the form of fat all around their body. Do you know many of you have willingly created a camel's hump on your belly because you're not drinking enough water? So, your belly is water retention and fat storage because you are not giving yourself enough water? If you want your liver and kidneys to work optimally, you must keep your hydration levels up.

Just some carbohydrates can lead to bloating.

This program raves about good carbohydrates – fruit, vegetables, salad, seeds, herbs and pulses. They are full of water. We blame the other type of carbohydrates for a lot of things. Still, when it comes to carbohydrates and water retention, the accusation is a fair one. Eating a diet high in sugary, starchy carbohydrates requires your body to store the extra calories. Because sugary carbohydrates cause an insulin spike and then a resulting drop in blood sugar, eating too many carbohydrates may keep you hungry and cause you to overeat. You can become a walking water balloon when you add salt into the mix — as with chips, crackers and French fries.

"I don't like water!"

Many people don't like water, so you are certainly not alone. Although over time, you get used to it. Would sparkling water be more attractive to you? If it is, there's no problem if you want to drink sparkling instead of still. Alternatively, have you tried water ice cold, hot or even room temperature? It's fascinating how many people discover that their enjoyment of water is very temperature dependent.

You could add flavour with a slice of cucumber, ginger or lemon, or a sprig of mint. Herbal teas are also excellent alternatives to plain water, so long as they don't contain caffeine and you don't add honey or sugar. So keep experimenting, and eventually, you'll find the combination that works best for you.

Caffeine

Sometimes a client will tell me that they have had 8 cups of tea instead of drinking water. Unfortunately, that doesn't count. In fact, caffeine is a diuretic, which means it's dehydrating. So for every cup of tea or coffee you drink, you need to have an extra glass of water to compensate. Caffeine is also one of the leading causes of cellulite, so most of us would prefer to avoid it. The liver can have problems processing too much coffee, so the body has to store that toxin somewhere. It can't store it around the organs as that would be dangerous, so instead, it simply stores it around the hip and thigh area – hence why lack of movement and excess coffee drinking has been proven to increase cellulite.

Caffeine is a fat burner. Green tea is excellent, but coffee or tea can make a difference. It's all about balance. One or two cups are enough to give you a fat-burning boost, wake you up in the morning or just let you enjoy a familiar mid-morning ritual. Any more than two cups a day, you start to see a negative impact on your health. Any caffeine after about 6 pm might also keep you awake at night.

Scientifically, it's been proven that one cup of tea or coffee can do your heart some good. It can boost it, and the arteries start to wake up. Don't forget that doesn't happen if you have milk in your coffee, though, as the milk kills that little boost before it even happens. However, once you're onto your second cup of coffee, that little adrenaline boost isn't so little. Adrenaline equals a signal that there might be a need for flight or fight – we are an animal. Therefore, the body might need to produce glucose for that flight or battle. By the next cup, there is far too much adrenaline in your body – adrenaline, therefore, begins to equal cortisol and glucose levels going up, ultimately driving fat storage.

I'm also going to suggest you try drinking your tea or coffee black or with just a splash of almond or soya milk. Many of my clients don't like this idea, and of course, it is your choice, but you might be surprised by how many of those people discover that they are happy to cut out the milk after just a few days. Like sugar addiction, milky drinks are a habit rather than a true addiction, so it only takes a few days to change.

There are several reasons to drink black or with just a little milk. First, we know that milk is not necessary from a nutritional point of view. Every nutrient in milk is also in the lovely food you eat. But milk is high in sugars and fats. If you have two milky coffees, like lattes or cappuccinos, every day, that milk adds up very quickly, and it will all sit around your belly as fat.

The other thing to remember is that a milky drink in the morning acts to break your fast. While we aren't doing intermittent fasting, we do want to allow autophagy to kick in. You also want to exercise before you eat when your cortisol level is low, and you will burn the fattest. Even if you don't eat breakfast until 10 am, you have broken your fast if you have a latte at 7 am. Autophagy will stop, and you'll burn blood sugar rather than fat when you exercise.

For that reason, if you choose to have a milky coffee, I suggest having it with breakfast after exercising. Stick to a splash of milk, black drinks or water first thing in the morning, and have an extra glass of water for every tea or coffee.

So, stick to a maximum of two caffeine's per day in the weight loss stage. Also, a clean fast is no tea or coffee at all – once you've had your tea or coffee at any point of the day, that puts you in a dirty fast mode, which might mean no fast. Again, all your choice entirely, of course. With my plan, there are no rules. You want to do the best you can for your health. I'm simply shining a light down a path you can choose. However, my clients determine the correct way to achieve outstanding results.

Best time to have your coffee

My suggestion below may solve all your questions regarding dirty fasts etc.

The best time to have your coffee is not right after waking up. Why? It involves the body's hormones, primarily cortisol. You might be familiar with cortisol as a stress hormone. Still, cortisol is the primary hormone from your adrenal gland that signals the body to be awake and responsive. Cortisol levels, which fluctuate throughout the day, typically peak in the morning – around 8:30 am.

However, caffeine increases the level of cortisol in the body. So, when you consume a cup of coffee within the first hour or two of waking, you are likely not getting caffeine's full benefits because your body is already at its peak cortisol level – trying to get you going. It is also thought that early morning caffeine might interfere with your normal morning cortisol production and stress your adrenal glands if you consume too much.

After cortisol peaks at around 8:30, it begins to decline, then spikes again around noon. So, 9:30 to 11:00 am might be the most advantageous window to benefit from your caffeine/coffee consumption. Although cortisol levels drop off again in the afternoon, that's probably not the best time for another coffee pickup because it could interfere with your sleep at the end of the day.

Green tea

Although green tea is caffeine, it has fantastic health benefits. You can reduce your caffeine intake to two caffeinated drinks daily and replace any others with green tea, which can significantly improve your health chances. Eventually, try eliminating all black teas and coffees and replacing all with green teas instead. You may be surprised how quickly your caffeine addiction will pass.

Just have a look at these comparisons….

Some facts about coffee:
- Caffeine
- 1000 chemical compounds
- adrenaline
- dopamine
- addiction

- bad breath
- toxins
- cellulite
- cortisol

Some facts about green tea:
- Caffeine
- antioxidants
- healthy bioactive compounds
- may improve brain function
- increases fat burning
- may lower the risk of some cancers
- may protect the brain from ageing
- may help prevent type 2 diabetes
- may help prevent cardiovascular disease

Herbal Teas

I often struggle with drinking 3 litres of water every day. If there is any part of this straightforward journey I battle with, it is the amount of water we should ingest. So, the simplest solution to keeping your hydration levels up without just water is by drinking herbal teas. Luckily there is a vast selection to help us with our cravings.

Alcohol

Alcohol is a big topic that deserves a chapter of its own, so I won't go into detail here. However, it's worth mentioning that alcohol dehydrates more than caffeine. Therefore, for every alcoholic drink, you will need two extra glasses of water to rehydrate yourself.

Fizzy Drinks

Diet Fizzy Drinks

Are fizzy drinks the answer if you don't like water and can't drink endless cups of tea? I used to think so. I drank huge amounts of Diet Coke; it has no sugar and calories, so it seemed like the perfect solution.

We now know that the aspartame in diet drinks is toxic, almost a poison. It causes many symptoms like nausea, cramps, mood swings, vision problems, fatigue and sleep disturbances. I've even heard of people under investigation for possible brain tumours - the symptoms went away when they gave up diet drinks. More commonly, they have a really gassy effect and can make you very bloated. I found that out for myself. I always had a bloated belly, no matter what I did. It went away when I stopped drinking Diet Coke, and I have never been bloated since.

Sweeteners can be up to 200 times sweeter than sugar. Think of one grain of sugar on a spoon the size of one sweetener, then imagine filling that spoon with 200 grains of sugar versus 200 sweetener tablets. You begin to see the picture! This amount of false sugar can make your body crave sugar or an insulin high even more than regular sugar, so diet drinks can lead to sugar cravings that could significantly impact our health journey.

You would be better off having a full-sugar drink. Or better still, avoid both!

Full Sugar Fizzy Drinks

One can of coke contains about 35g of sugar or 8 teaspoons. All that sugar will shoot straight into your bloodstream and send your blood sugar sky high, with the inevitable crash later. So it just feeds the sugar addiction.

Fizzy drinks have no beneficial nutrients, fibre, vitamins or minerals. They are entirely pointless, and they really are killing us. Many of my clients drink fizzy drinks before they come to me, and when they stop, they find that all sorts of poor health conditions go away. Things like IBS, bloating, acid reflux and diarrhoea are all gone just by giving up fizzy drinks. So is it worth putting that in your body? All you need in life is water, herbal teas if you like them and a couple of cups of caffeine as an optional extra.

The joy is how easy it is to give up these fizzy drinks. Literally just 3 days! Time and time again, I have had clients terrified at going cold turkey off their fizzy drinks. Some clients are on as many as eight per day. But I can promise you that my clients receive the same beautiful results every time. They miss the drinks a lot on day one and day two, but by day three, they feel it's like a miracle. They are amazed that they don't miss them anymore. Sugar addiction is a three-day elimination process to get to the holy grail; being a sugar addict no longer.

Milk

The milk industry, especially alternative "milk", is an interesting example of marketing and consumerism over health. We are constantly bombarded with messages telling us that various types of milk are good for us. Oats, nuts, and even peas are used to make milk substitutes and are sold as healthy options. They may be helpful products for vegans or people who have allergies, but they are certainly not healthy drinks.

This marketing includes animal milk. We are told that milk is essential for bone health when the truth is that you will get all the calcium you need from pulses, soy and green vegetables. As an adult, you don't have to drink any milk. Lactose is fat, a carb, and a protein which is, therefore, a drink only needed for a baby not yet eating. Once you are eating foods for your nutrition, why would you need lactose again? A serving of lactose milk can be 3 teaspoons of processed sugar. No animal in the wild is sucking off other animals' nipples once it's weaned. So why do humans continue drinking cow's milk? Maybe we need to ask the milk marketing lobbyist that?

Just a reminder of sugar levels in 1 cup (240 ml) of various types of unsweetened milk
- Cow's milk (whole and skim): 12 grams
- Rice milk: 13 grams
- Soy milk: 1 gram
- Oat milk: 5 grams
- Coconut milk: 3 grams
- Almond milk: 0 grams

I'm not saying you should give up all milk forever, but making an informed choice is essential.

Oat and Rice milks

Beware of trendy marketing encouraging you to eat or drink completely unnecessary sugars! Oat milk is a favourite now. Many people are consuming oat milk lattes and feeling that they are being healthy. The opposite is true. We aren't counting calories, but an oat milk latte can be a whopping 220 calories. Pour that amount of milk into a jug 365 days a year, and then imagine all those jugs in a row, all storing fat around your belly. One oat milk latte a day for a year equals 80,300 calories of sugar!

If you think about it, oats are a high-GI food. This is because they are pure carbohydrates, and oat milk is effectively sugar. In fact, that oat latte contains 23g of sugar - 6 teaspoons total. The same applies to rice milks or any other milk made from a complex grain carbohydrate. They are little more than sugar water. You might also like to know that the "barista" milk blends, formulated to make perfect cappuccinos and lattes, add quite a lot of fat.

Nut milks

At the other end of the scale, we have nut milks, the most common being almond. Nuts are a protein to feed your brain and body. An almond milk latte is 73 calories, a third of the oat milk version. As we know, nuts are not perfect for the weight loss stage. Still, if you want an occasional latte, almond milk has far less fat, sugar and calories than oat milk and would be a much better choice. Remember, a latte is instead of breakfast, not in addition too.

Soya milk

Soya milk is a very healthy option if you do want to have milk. Soya is full of many good things, like potassium, vitamin D and iron. It's also a great source of protein, so this would be my preferred option if you don't want to drink your tea and coffee black. A soya milk latte, for example, could be consumed **instead** of breakfast on an odd day. This is an 'instead of' rather than an 'as well as'. For example, suppose you're travelling and find the only available outlet is a Café Nero or Starbucks, where everything is starchy carbohydrates. In that case, soya milk is an excellent way of having a hefty dose of protein/carbs rather than going down the starchy food route.

Coconut milk

If you were running around naked on a desert island with little to eat, you would need concentrated, high-energy food to keep you going. Coconut would be perfect. Full of fats, carbohydrates and sugars. As it is, you don't live on a desert island, you're probably not running around all day, and you have plenty of other foods to enjoy, so you don't need all those fats and sugars during the weight management stage.

Cow's Milk

Whole milk is full of creamy fat. But, on the other hand, a whole milk latte contains roughly the same energy as two and a half lovely fluffy scrambled eggs. So I know which one I would tuck into instead!

Skimmed milk isn't any better than milk either. Of course, the fat is removed during manufacture and to make the milk palatable, they replace it with sugar. This makes skimmed milk another high-sugar option.

Ideally, you will have your coffee black or with a dash of milk, but if you want a latte with your breakfast, then the best choices are soya or almond milk. Be aware that some brands blend different types of milk if you are buying a carton to use at home. For example, your "almond milk" might be combined with rice milk, which is cheaper for the manufacturer. It's always worth checking the labels.

Juices, Smoothies & Soups: eat it, don't juice it.

Apple juice has 500 calories per carton
Orange juice has 500 calories per carton

Imagine I gave you a huge bowl piled high with strawberries. Next to it are three big oranges. Could you eat it all? Possibly not! It would take quite a long time to munch your way through, with lots of chewing (which signals to your brain that you have eaten) and fibre to help your digestive system work well. You would have to focus on what you were doing, choose which strawberry to eat next and concentrate on peeling the oranges. How would you feel at the end? Probably full.

If you took the same fruits and made them into juice, you would only get a small glass, which you would probably down in seconds. With no fibre, there is nothing to chew, nothing to fill you up or signal to your brain that you have "eaten". How would you feel after a small glass of juice? Still hungry? Most people have juice alongside other foods because a drink doesn't feel like enough.

You have essentially turned your fruit into strawberry-flavoured sugar water. It doesn't satisfy you and sends your blood sugar shooting up - feeding your sugar addiction.

On top of that, since juice doesn't feel like a meal, most people will also eat something else and use milk or yoghurt as ingredients in a smoothie. Remember that mixing fruit with other foods, especially dairy foods, inhibits the absorption of essential vitamins and minerals.

How many spoons of sugar are in orange juice?

6 teaspoons. Orange Juice – 24g (**6 teaspoons**) of sugar per 8oz of juice, meaning a small 8 oz. glass of orange juice has the equivalent of 4 oranges.

How many spoons of sugar are in apple juice?

For example, 12 ounces of 100% apple juice, a standard portion size, contains **10 teaspoons** of sugar – the same amount found in a 12-ounce Coca-Cola. The same portion of orange juice includes nine teaspoons, while grape juice contains a whopping 15 teaspoons of sugar.

To get the health benefits of eating your fruit, don't drink it. Instead, always have it raw at least two hours after a meal.

Eat it, don't soup it.

There's an interesting quirk of human biology: hot foods fill you up more than cold foods. This is because something about the temperature registers with your brain and helps to trigger the satiety mechanism. That's one of the reasons why I recommend a hot lunch, especially in winter.

Many people immediately turn to soup. First, however, you need to be aware of potential pitfalls.

First, nearly all ready-made soups are made with many cheap fillers - even the high-end fresh ones. Check the list on the packet; you will usually see potatoes or rice as one of the main ingredients. If you want to eat soup, you will almost certainly have to make your own to avoid these high GI grains or root vegetables.

When your body starts preparing to eat, the saliva is stimulated, which forms the chemical processes your body needs to undergo for successful digestion. When you chew your food, your body goes through mastication and peristalsis to move the food through the digestive tract. This results in food eventually reaching the cells as it should and fibre being produced to help with the whole process. When you soup your food, what do you get? Just sugar water, no mastication, no peristalsis, and much-reduced fibre. That's why I always say – eat it, don't soup it!

If your soup is blended, especially on the thinner side, it is effectively just hot vegetable juice. Just like fruit juice, it's sugar water. Your soup will feed your sugar addiction and leave you feeling hungry. There's a reason it's traditionally served with bread - you need something to fill you up!

You can make a soup to help you in the weight loss journey. Use ingredients like pulses, proteins and vegetables and make it a soup you can chew. Something that you eat, not drink.

Detoxes

Have you ever been tempted by those detox programs? Perhaps even one where you get to spend a week or two in a luxury resort somewhere beautiful, living on juices or soups and doing yoga on the beach every day? They certainly sound enticing, with a price tag to match!

While there's nothing wrong with relaxing, the idea of a juice detox is ultimately flawed. You have cut out all the main food groups, so, you lose weight. Anyone would, but all that changes as soon as you go home. After spending a week living on sugar water, your body is utterly confused and thinks you are at risk of starvation. As soon as you start eating normally, your body will grab the opportunity to lay down stores in case of a famine, and you will gain more weight than you lost.

Have you ever experienced that? You have some success with whatever the latest fad diet is, but as soon as you stop, all the weight piles back on. That's why it's essential to understand that this is not a diet. It's not a one-week detox or even a six-month plan. We don't cut out food groups or do anything unsustainable. This is about crafting your new lifestyle and supporting your health for the rest of your life.

Yasmin, David and Sophie

Yasmin

Yasmin used to follow all sorts of "wellness influencers" on Instagram, and she got sick and tired of all the wheatgrass juices and detox programs they always seemed to be on. She remembers how she would always feel jealous of their pictures, glass in hand, in some exotic location. Still, when she tried to recreate that at home, she was always left feeling hungry, exhausted and depressed as she battled acne and weight gain in rainy London.

Yasmin has just been through and unfollowed every one of those Instagram accounts, and she feels like a huge weight has been lifted from her shoulders. (She has also followed me @theweightlossgurucom for more realistic inspiration!)

David

David will admit that he likes a latte, preferably with toffee syrup. Especially when he's on a long night shift in the ambulance, and the drive-through gives paramedics free drinks. At that time of night, he can't go anywhere for a soy latte, and his colleagues like the current drive-through anyway, so David will try a two-pronged approach.

He will bring a large bottle of water throughout his shift (with a squeeze of lemon - he hates it plain). Then, when everyone else gets lattes, he will have a black coffee or an americano with a tiny splash of milk and no sugar. David has even told his colleagues his plan so that he has accountability and won't change his mind in a moment of weakness at 2 am.

Sophie

Sophie spends her days busily dashing from one thing to the next, heating up the same cold cup of coffee 5 times in the microwave without drinking a drop. She could quickly get to 5 pm without drinking anything sometimes.

Her focus for the next few days is to drink a glass of water every hour. She has a smartwatch and has set it to chime every hour between 7 am and 7 pm not an annoying alarm, but just a gentle reminder. Sophie has also dug out a water bottle with a sports cap. She thinks she'll be more likely to drink water if she can put it down without worrying about the baby knocking her cup over!

Over to You

Grab your journal or iPhone and make plans for the next week. Remember, you don't have to do everything at once. If it feels like a lot, choose one small step for this week and build on it next week. Here are some things you might want to think about:

How will I make sure I drink enough water?

Will I have any caffeine drinks, and if so, when?

Will I switch to a different milk, or try drinks black?

Do I need to make any other changes, like giving up juice, buying some herbal tea or making soup?

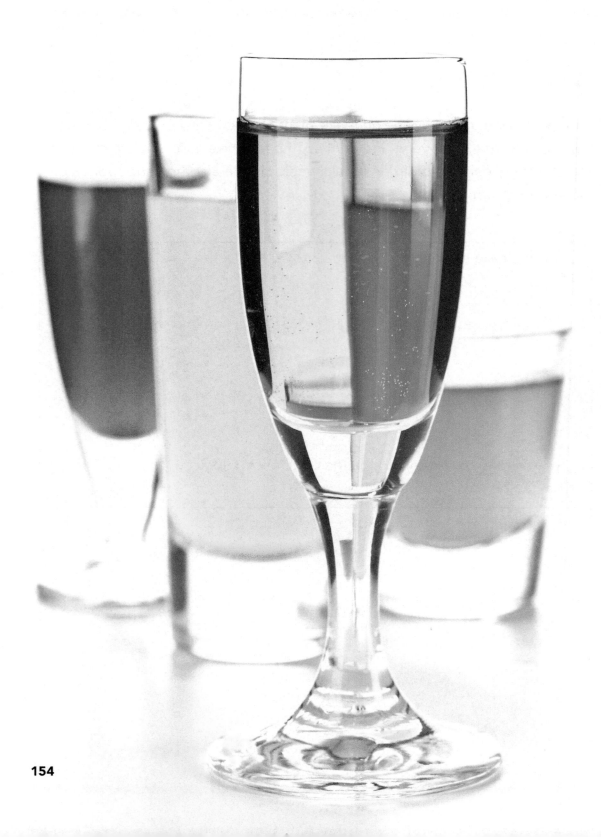

154

A - Alcohol

"If you want to turn a vision into reality, you must give 100% and never stop believing in your dream." - Arnold Schwarzenegger

Here we are at step five of the seven simple steps. So far, we have looked at which foods and drinks will help you reach your goals and how to cut out the junk. We've considered the best time to eat as well. So, you know what you want to put into your body but knowing that and doing it are two different things! We will look at the emotional and psychological sides in the next chapters, but let's focus on one of the main ways people trip up - alcohol.

It might seem a bit extreme to devote a whole chapter to alcohol, but the truth is that it is that important in your weight loss journey. Alcohol affects you both psychologically and physically, so the potential impact on your health is enormous. But, of course, our main aim is always better health. That's why I'm going to devote a whole chapter to giving you the information you need to make wise choices regarding "wine o'clock" or Friday night drinks.

What is Alcohol?

What do you think alcohol is? A carbohydrate, fat or protein? In fact, alcohol is quite unique in that it's none of them. It's a toxin! It's not a macronutrient or a micronutrient. It contains no vitamins or minerals. Nothing to add to your diet except empty calories.

We already know that carbohydrates and proteins are 4 calories per gram, and fats are 9 calories per gram. Alcohol comes in at 7 calories per gram. So, when you drink alcohol, it's almost like pouring melted cheese down your throat! Of course, calories aren't everything, but even so, it is a clue as to why drinking lots of alcohol is not ideal in the weight loss phase.

Do you remember in chapter 1 that I told you that the body you live in is almost entirely your creation? 80% of it has been created by what you eat, 15% by the exercise you have done, and the last 5% is genetics. Alcohol significantly impacts your health. If you drink a lot of alcohol, those proportions change. Your body becomes 60% what you drink, 20% what you eat, 15% exercise and 5% genetics.

At 7 calories per gram, alcohol will affect your weight, but that's not all. It affects your health, your lifestyle, your mental health - everything!

"Do I have to go tee-total?"

Of course not! I'm not going to tell you to give up alcohol entirely because this is a lifestyle, not a short-term diet. If you try to restrict yourself too much, you won't be able to sustain that change. Instead, you'll have a hard day, get in a bad mood, and rebel. Instead of a restrictive, short-term diet, we need a lifestyle change that you can stick with for life, a way for weight to fall away and stay gone - forever.

We live in a culture where it's considered normal to drink most days, perhaps a glass of wine after work and another with dinner. A bit more on Friday or Saturday. It's entirely understandable if you follow that pattern, but it's not helping you to reach your goals. Could you cut down and drink no more than 2 units of alcohol on just two nights a week?

I have a client who lost 39kg by cutting back on alcohol. She used to drink five nights a week and cut that down to one night. That's it, she didn't change her food at all, but she lost a considerable amount of weight. So 39kg, gone forever! That could be you.

Alcohol and Calories

Of course, there is more to healthy eating than calories, but they can be a helpful shorthand to help you understand what's happening when you have "just a few" drinks.

Obviously, some alcoholic drinks contain far more calories than others. For example, anything containing cream or a lot of sugar will be far higher. For the sake of illustration, we can say that a unit of alcohol typically averages around 100 calories.

The first thing to be aware of is how rarely we have just one unit of alcohol. A glass of red wine at home is very often three units. So that's 300 calories per glass. Let's say you come in from a hard day at work and pour a glass of wine, which you sip while you unwind from the day and start cooking supper. When the meal is ready, your glass is empty (how did that happen?), so you fill it back up. Just one drink with your meal, which you tell yourself is pretty restrained. Then you settle down to watch a movie, and it would only be movie night with a glass of wine. You deserve it after the day you've had!

That is a typical scenario, the sort of thing that millions of people do every day. But you have just consumed 900 extra calories. That's the same as nine chocolate bars! Not only that, but you also should have noticed doing it.

Let's look at it another way. How much wine do you drink in a week? Maybe a bottle? For many people, that's only one bottle of wine weekly. Over a year, though, it adds up to about 30,000 calories. The same as eating a Big Mac every week. Do you drink more than that? Two bottles a week? Or three? The calories add up fast.

Only some people drink wine, so we'll also have a look at beer. One pint of beer is about 200 calories, equivalent to two packets of crisps. How many pints might you have in an evening at the pub? By the time everyone has bought a round, it might be quite a few! You could quickly be drinking the calorie equivalent of 8 or 10 packets of crisps - not to mention the bar snacks that might tempt you as well. Remember, these are empty calories with no beneficial nutrients at all. No protein, carbohydrates or even fat. No vitamins or minerals. Nothing that your body needs. Alcohol is also a toxin. It stops your metabolism from burning carbs and fats, and you won't burn any fat for two days after drinking it!

Let's say you have three large glasses of wine on a Wednesday, 900 empty calories. That alcohol then sits on your liver, stopping your metabolism until Friday. Then you can celebrate the weekend with another drink! You can see that losing weight is impossible if you drink every night or even every other night. Your liver is your fat burner, and so long as you keep drinking regularly, you will never allow it to get rid of those toxins and you'll get stuck in the weight loss process. On the other hand, if you cut down and only drink at the weekend (for example), you have five days left for weight loss. It's a dramatic difference.

Alcohol's Impact on Health

Leaky Gut Syndrome

Protein, carbohydrates, and fats go into your gut when you eat foods. You swallow them, and they enter your digestive system, where they are meant to be.

Believe it, that is not what happens when you drink beer! As a toxin, beer has no place in your gut, so it leaks out. It slowly seeps out of your gut, and from there, it washes around your other organs. Of course, everything that is in beer goes too, not just alcohol but also wheat, hops and malt. A study in America found that 100% of the beer drinkers they tested had leaky gut syndrome. Every single one.

This may be a little graphic, but you need to understand. The wheat, malt and hops, having leaked out of your gut, have entered your liver and kidneys. They are not meant to be in your body, and your body and organs don't know how to process them, so they hang around. Pretty soon, they start to develop a fungus and then parasites. Yes, you read that right. If you use a microscope to look at a tissue sample from someone who drinks a lot of beer, you will find parasites in their body.

Not what we want for optimum health! Wine doesn't contain wheat or hops as beer does, but it is acidic. Like beer, it is not a micro or a macronutrient, so it has no place to go once it's in your body. Instead, it leaks out of your gut, and all that acid gets into your kidney and liver. Remember that your liver is your fat burner, so anything stopping it from doing its job will impact your weight loss and health.

Sleep

We all know that alcohol impacts our sleep. After a "heavy" drinking session of 6 units (or just 2 of those large glasses of wine), you will wake up more often to go to the loo, for example. But it goes deeper than that. Did you know that alcohol also changes the nature of your sleep? It disrupts your sleep cycles.

This is a problem for two main reasons. Firstly, your body simply isn't getting the rest it needs. It's awake for much of the night, so it isn't burning fat the way it usually would.

The second problem is what happens the next day. You wake up tired, exhausted even, and perhaps hungover. So, you do what we all do when we're tired - grab something to give you energy. Unfortunately, you almost certainly reach for the wrong thing - sugar. You have a temporary sugar high, but soon you crash again and start looking for something else. Up and down, all day long, eating more and more sugar.

Mental Health

I have noticed an interesting trend among my clients. Quite a few come to me after experiencing cancer. They have been through treatment and are now cancer-free. Typically, they don't worry about cancer coming back. But when they drink, they worry. Repeatedly clients have told me that the day after they drink alcohol, they feel paranoid that their cancer might return.

The link between alcohol and mental health is well established, and we know it's a vicious cycle. Alcohol makes you feel depressed, and being depressed makes you reach for alcohol. Round and round, in ever-decreasing spirals. The only solution is to break the cycle.

When people are treated for depression, they are usually told to stop drinking. In alcohol addiction clinics, patients are treated for depression. They go hand in hand, which means that if you reduce the amount you drink, you will almost certainly be happier for it.

Self-Control

There you are, following the plan, doing well. You've dropped a few kgs, look and feel great, and decide to celebrate. What happens after a few drinks? You lose all self-control. Willpower goes out the window, and before you know it, you are ordering that sugary, fatty pudding and devouring it as if your life depended on it. And you don't stop there either!

Did you know that alcohol lowers your levels of leptin, the satiety hormone? Leptin regulates your appetite. When it's high, you feel full, and when it's low, you feel hungry. So since alcohol causes low leptin, it makes you feel hungry. No wonder so many people stop for a kebab on the way home!

The impact of alcohol isn't just about the calories in your drinks and the fact that it sits on your liver for days. It's also about the extra foods you eat when you drink, the bread, fried foods and sugar you reach for to "help" with a hangover and tiredness the next day. But, really, it's a three-day process to get back to burning fat the way you want to.

If you struggle to cut down

It can be challenging to cut down on alcohol for all sorts of reasons. Social pressure and the force of habit are genuine and can cause cravings that are hard to resist. Of course, we can't ignore the possibility of addiction. If you are struggling, you will find some tools in the next chapter that can help you curb cravings for alcohol just as well as they can be used to cut down on food.

If you know my story, you'll see that I have family experience with alcoholism. I take alcohol seriously because I have seen how it can impact you and those around you. If you feel that your mental health is severely affected by alcohol or struggle to reduce your drinking amount, please consider seeking extra help. You can turn many places, from your doctor to local AA meetings.

Please reach out to someone.

Alcohol and Hunger

Very often, when people feel they need a drink, they are hungry. My clients often tell me that at about 5 or 6pm, they "need" a drink. We already know that humans need to eat about every four hours, so if you had lunch at 1 or 2pm, you're hungry by 6pm! Your blood sugar is low, and you genuinely crave something to keep you going. The strange thing is wouldn't it just be easier to eat dinner at 6pm - easier and healthier! We live in a system where we're told it's too early. We've got used to eating at 9pm and using alcohol to get past our natural 6pm hunger. Of course, eating so late, we go to bed with a full belly and don't burn fat the way we should. It all makes so much sense when you put it together!

If you need a drink at 5 or 6pm, can you eat dinner instead? As you saw in chapter 4, that's when you should really be eating dinner anyway. The added advantage is that when you satisfy your hunger, you may not need alcohol in the evenings at all.

What to Drink

Alcohol

Hopefully, by now, I have convinced you to drink on just two nights a week, so the next question is what to have. You now know that beer gives you parasites, so you may want to avoid it. Not only that, but wine is also very acidic, especially white wine, and that is why it gives you such a bad headache and can make you feel very ill. There is also the danger that once you open a bottle of wine, your glass keeps getting topped up, and you lose all sense of how much you have had. Luckily, there are better choices out there!

The best drinks for weight loss are highly distilled and transparent. Let's start with gin. One shot of gin is still 100 calories, but it's a less acidic drink with no sugar. Have your gin with tonic if you want but avoid low calorie, sugar-free or slimline. That usually means sweetener has been added and is to be avoided at all costs as seen in previous chapters. If you are going to reduce your alcoholic intake significantly then make sure you enjoy the few drinks you do have. Have it with *Fever Tree* tonic (or whatever you love) so you don't feel restricted or deprived. If you don't like gin, then some other good options are rum and tequila.

Vodka is an interesting one. Some brands are made from grapes, which makes them better. The most popular brands, though, tend to be made from wheat. That takes us back to the fungus, mould and parasites we get from beer, so vodka is only sometimes a good choice. Some are made from potato, milk or cheese, which are all less than ideal. If you like vodka, always check and get to know your brands.

Another advantage of drinking spirits is that it puts you in control. When you go out to dinner, and everyone shares a few bottles of wine, people are constantly topping up each other's glasses. Often, they don't even ask! That makes it impossible to know how much you've had, and you must spend the whole evening putting your hand over your glass and saying "no", which can get tedious, if not embarrassing. With spirits, nobody can top your glass up. You know exactly how much you've had. Most often, people will not offer to buy you more as spirits are so expensive, so you won't have to reject them. In addition, nobody will ever notice if you swap to a non-alcoholic drink, plain tonic or even water.

Non-alcoholic Alternatives

Are you shuddering at the thought of the alcohol-free lager we had years ago? Alcohol-free drinks used to be nasty. You were left with a choice between sugary fizzy drinks (not very sophisticated in a high-end restaurant, and not good for you) or water. There are so many more options available, many of which are good.

One of my favourites is Seedlip, which you can check out at seedlipdrinks. com. They are a British company that makes non-alcoholic distilled drinks as an alternative to spirits. Seedlip comes in three flavours, and my favourite is the citrus "Grove 42", which tastes just like gin. You can order Seedlip in restaurants and many bars now, and of course, you can keep it at home as well (ordering online is much cheaper). They even sell pre-mixed cans of Seedlip and tonic.

Tanqueray alcohol-free gin is fantastic as well. Serve it with your favourite Fever Tree tonic, and I challenge you to tell the difference. Gordons Alcohol-Free Premium Pink Gin is another excellent option – there are so many to choose from! There are also now some divine alcohol free champagnes, proseccos and red wines out there. The champagne I recommend is Wild Idol. Honestly, you can't tell the difference if it contains alcohol or not!

For many clients it's not the alcohol that they actually need at the end of a stressful day or week. It's just the ritual. So sit with you favourite drink -non alcohol this time - in your favourite chair with your favourite glass and ice and lemon and I challenge you to see that it's not the alcohol you need. It's the experience, the winding down, the moment, the ritual. You'll feel just as good but with non of the negative consequences!

The Social Side

Do you worry that people will think you're boring if you don't drink? When we socialise, we are not there for alcohol. We are there to enjoy spending time with family or friends, eat good food, soak up the atmosphere and enjoy an event. We don't have to rely on alcohol to have fun. It comes from so many other aspects of a night out.

Honestly, the most interesting people are those who don't need to rely on alcohol to enjoy a social event. They are the people with the most to say, the ones you can have fascinating conversations with. Drunk people (or even slightly tipsy people) are often the boring ones! If you're angry, alcohol can make you angrier and even more annoyed with your spouse. You become more aggravated, feeling down you feel even worse. We want to find the positives in life, not increase the negatives.

Nobody pays attention to what you order at a restaurant unless you fuss about it. You can easily order anything you want, one gin and tonic followed by Seedlip or water. Everyone will be so busy chatting and thinking about their orders that they won't even notice.

If anyone does ask, you can say that you aren't drinking today. Tell your friends that you're aiming to lose weight, you're on antibiotics, driving, or whatever you feel comfortable saying. Does it really matter? Why would they care whether you drink?

A Little Challenge

I have a challenge for you. One night this week, when you will be out with friends, and there will be social pressure to drink, don't have any alcohol. Before you go, get out your phone or journal and make some notes. What is likely to happen that will make you want to drink? What situations will you encounter, or what things might people say? What will you do instead?

For example:

- My friend has big news and will probably buy champagne to celebrate. I will bring a bottle of Noughty or Nozeco and have a glass of that instead.

- If someone offers me a drink, I'll say I'm driving.

- If my favourite cocktail is on the menu, I'll remember that while I enjoy the drink, I don't like the hangover, and I'll try a new mocktail instead.

- If someone gets bolshy and says I'm being boring, I'll say I don't need to drink to be fun.

The next day makes some more notes in your iPhone or journal. How did people react, and how did you feel about it? Did you enjoy your evening? How do you feel waking up the following day? Do you want to do it again?

For more tips on making this happen, and using the RAIN model to make changes, look at chapter 8.

The Big Experiment

Are you truly serious about losing weight? Really and truly committed to changing your life forever and becoming healthy, slim and happy? If so, I would like to suggest an experiment. Why not try drinking no alcohol at all, just for the next three weeks? Then, when the three weeks are up, see how you feel. If you want to start drinking one or two nights a week, go ahead. It's your choice. But you may find that you don't want to.

When my clients try this experiment, they are almost always surprised, and even shocked, by how good they feel. They love being clear-headed, with no hangovers, better skin, more energy - and weight loss. As a result, they want to refrain from going back to drinking regularly. Try it. Maybe you'll love the results too!

Alcohol Addiction Quiz

This is a quiz I like to do with my clients so we can discuss which, if any, of these situations you might have a predetermined emotional issue with. We then examine your relationship with each situation and why and where that comes from initially. Then, we devise a plan that will change lifetime habits. You can't ever just become a different person. You can't just suddenly decide to change your personality. That's not possible. It would help if you made an actual plan, a physical strategy that means you make conscious, material changes to your daily routine. Suggest what or how you will substitute, choose, replace, strategise now you see the way to a lighter life.

For Example:
- Say you are driving
- Set the number of evenings
- Go out less
- Plan how many evenings you will drink per week in a diary
- Go for zero-alcohol drinks
- Go for spirits over wine/beer
- Choose a really filling fish, chicken, or vegan dish and use STOP when ordering
- Assess your 'purpose' before you go
- Listen to RAIN before you go

Let's say that heroin refers to alcohol and sawdust refers to bread and pasta ... because nutritionally they offer the same thing!

1. Could you happily go out to the theatre and not have heroin or sawdust the entire evening? What would you have instead? Plan a new strategy.

2. Could you happily go out to a sports evening, such as football or tennis, and not have heroin or sawdust the entire match? What would you have instead? Plan a new strategy.

3. Could you happily go out for dinner with a friend or friends and not have heroin or sawdust the entire evening? What would you have instead? Plan a new strategy.

4. Could you happily go out to a friend's party or wedding and not have heroin or sawdust the entire evening? What would you have instead? Plan a new strategy.

5. Could you happily go to a work event and not have heroin or sawdust the entire evening? What would you have instead? Plan a new strategy.

Yasmin, David and Sophie

Yasmin

Yasmin loves going out with her friends for cocktails and sometimes karaoke. But she doesn't love the hangovers so much! So she tried one alcohol-free night out, switching to mocktails, and loved waking up the next day with a clear head.

Yasmin's first thought was to switch to mocktails long term. Still, those tend to have a lot of sugar, so she will try Seedlip and tonic instead and a couple of cocktails on Friday nights. She might even see if she can drag her friends onto the dancefloor more often, and they may drink a little less.

David

David has always been a fan of a beer or two in front of the football or a few beers when everyone starts getting rounds in at the pub. He was horrified to read about the leaky gut syndrome and hasn't had a beer since. His mates might tease him about his "G and T", but he doesn't want fungus and parasites! It's also a lot easier to stick to just the two drinks.

On non-drinking days he has started telling everyone he's on call for work. Maybe he takes his car and must stay sober to drive home. Nobody ever questions it.

Sophie

Sophie is getting sucked into the "Mummy's wine time" culture. She feels solidarity with other mums as they all seem to count down until bedtime to pour that first glass. Looking back, she doesn't know how it became a daily habit, except that parenting can be difficult, and she felt like she needed some reward.

Sophie has never enjoyed spirits, so she plans to try some alcohol-free wines and stop drinking altogether. She's excited to start with the three-week experiment and see if she feels any differently. She's also going to look for other ways to treat herself. For example, a new hobby could be her way to relax and something to look forward to when everyone is in bed.

Over to You

Are you ready to make a change? Will you take on one of the challenges? Get out your iPhone or journal to record your plans. Here are a few things to think about.

The One Night Challenge
I will try this challenge on (date):

Things that will tempt me to drink:

How I will avoid temptation:

How I feel afterwards:

The Three-Week Experiment
I will start this experiment on (date):

Things that might tempt me to drink:

How I will avoid temptation:

How I feel after the experiment:

My plan moving forwards (Stay alcohol-free? Drink? How many times a week?):

My Alcoholic Drinks

Next week I will drink on these days:

I will have these drinks:

After I have had two units of alcohol I will switch to:

Avoiding Alcohol

These are the non-alcoholic drinks that I want to try:

Things I will do instead of drinking (have dinner early, go for a walk, start a new hobby):

This person will be my cheerleader; I'll tell them my plans and ask them to support me.

I – Investigate Emotional Eating

"The most important thing is to enjoy your life - to be happy - it's all that matters." - Steve Jobs

Everything we have done so far is the easy part. Anyone can learn about healthy foods or find out what time to eat. Anyone can be told the dangers of alcohol. The trouble is that more than simply having that knowledge is needed. You must put it into practice every day.

Most of us have had the experience of carefully following some food plan, everything going well until *something* happens. It might be a big celebration, with champagne and cake. But, on the other hand, it could be a stressful day that sends you to the freezer in search of ice cream. Perhaps a particular relative that you can't say no to or a favourite bakery you can only walk past if you go inside. Whatever it is, something throws you off track, and you struggle to recover.

This is not a diet to follow religiously, but it is a lifestyle change, and any change can be challenging at first. In this chapter, I want to equip you with techniques to help you understand yourself and your deeper motivations and be prepared to handle those challenging moments confidently. Of course, you may enjoy a little birthday cake. That's your choice. The important thing is that you made a choice from a place of understanding, and you know what to do next.

Your Relationship with Food

The fact that you have bought this book suggests that you need more than simple instruction in nutrition. For example, most people who are overweight know that vegetables are healthier than cake. Of course, that's an oversimplification, but you see where I'm coming from. If nutritional information was all people needed to lose weight - nobody would ever be heavier than they wanted to be.

The truth is that we are not robots. We are gloriously complicated humans who don't always behave as cold logic suggests. The fact that you have gained more weight than you would like indicates that you have a distorted relationship with food. There are many possibilities, but the most likely is sugar addiction and/or an emotional eating issue.

If you don't address this, it doesn't matter how much you know about nutrition. You can have everything in place to eat for health, but you will still eat more significant portions than you need, eat at the wrong times and eat bad foods.

The Solution Bar?

Before we go any further, I would like you to do an exercise with me. It's straightforward, but it can reveal quite a lot.

Imagine that I have just handed you a brand-new invention. I'm over the moon to share this with you. It's the cutting edge of science. The solution bar contains all the nutrients you need for a day. All the macronutrients and all the micronutrients are carefully worked out for your exact needs by scientists. All you must do is eat one bar once a day. You will never have to worry about cooking, shopping, or meal planning again. You will lose weight steadily, and once you reach your goal, you will maintain that weight effortlessly. 7 bars will be delivered to your house every week for the rest of your life; that is all you will ever need to eat.

How do you feel? Suppose you are ready to place your order right now with not the slightest hesitation. In that case, it's safe to say that you don't have a food addiction or emotional eating issue. You see the bar as the ultimate solution, freeing you up to focus on family, hobbies, travel, building your business and everything else. You have food entirely in its place as fuel. Feel free to move on to the next chapter. Only a few people would fall into that category, though!

You don't feel 100% joyful at the thought of never eating anything other than the solution bar for the rest of your life. Why not? What was your first thought, your initial reaction? Did you think that you would miss the social side of eating out? Would you happily give up everything except chocolate (pasta or bread)? Do you enjoy cooking to shower your family and friends with love? Do you think that you'll never enjoy a Saturday evening again? Are you worrying that there is no point to Christmas or birthday's ever again because the whole reason for celebrating anything is to eat and drink? Do you think you'll have no excuse not to go for that promotion if you're thin?

There is no correct answer here, but your gut reaction to the solution bar gives you some interesting clues about your relationship with food. It's worth sitting with this for a while, perhaps journaling about it to see what comes up.

Sugar Addiction

We have discussed sugar addiction before, but it's worth mentioning again. Sugar, in this context, does not mean sweets and puddings. It means all complex carbohydrates - high GI foods like pasta, bread and potatoes. These foods are great if you are a farmer or hunter, requiring lots of energy during the day. When you eat those foods, they raise your blood sugar dramatically. This causes your body to flood with dopamine first, followed by insulin as it tries to deal with the excess by storing it as fat. Ultimately it leaves you gaining weight and feeling hungry, tired, bloated and depressed.

The good news is that if you can cut out that junk and eat foods that support your body, you will feel much healthier almost from the first day. Not only that, but your excess weight will also fall away, almost as a side effect of your newfound health and well-being.

Could you be a sugar addict? I am not only talking about the person who has a dessert after every meal, spoonful of sugar in their coffee and a stash of chocolates "for the grandchildren". Sugar addiction is far more insidious than that.

A sugar addict might have a glass of orange juice and a bowl of porridge for breakfast, a biscuit with "elevenses", and a sandwich for lunch. Starting the day with a sugar hit like juice and cereal sets you up for a mid-morning crash, so you begin drip-feeding more sugar. You are always trying to stay ahead of the next crash by eating more and more. If you think of a typical diet, it's probably more common to be a sugar addict than not in our culture. Eating sugars with meals and snacks is considered normal and even encouraged.

Breaking sugar addiction is, thankfully, very easy. When you eat sugar, you crave it. Your neurotransmitters are crying out for more sugar! But if you avoid sugar, it only takes a couple of days for those cravings to disappear completely. Unlike a true addiction, there is no withdrawal very little chemical addiction to break free from. As soon as the sugar is out of your system, you simply no longer need it, and within a few days, you won't believe that you ever did. All that is left then is a habit and any emotional eating issues.

Food Addictions

Food addiction must be the most common addiction on the planet. Before a baby can even lift their head, it can demand to be fed or refuse to eat. It's the only thing they have any power over. Unfortunately, for some people, that feeling lasts, or perhaps it's triggered again during childhood or even later.

If you felt that the solution bar would ruin your life, you might be a food addict. You might have thought that food is your one true pleasure, that you get through the day by dreaming of the delicious dinner waiting for you at home. You may start planning each meal before you have eaten the previous one. Food is always on your mind. Don't worry if you think you are addicted to food. I promise that you are not the only one, and the strategies in this chapter will help you.

Emotional Eating

Did you feel like the solution bar would spoil birthdays and Christmases? How could you celebrate without food? How would you cheer yourself up after a bad day or relax when stressed? If food is the thing you turn to when you have any strong emotions, then you may have an emotional eating issue. This is very common, so it's nothing to feel ashamed of, but if you don't address it, you will struggle to lose weight and be as healthy as you want.

How much happiness does it give you if you eat a chocolate bar because you feel sad? Two minutes? Five, if you eat slowly. What happens after that? Chocolate doesn't solve whatever problem you're facing. It can't take away the painful emotions. In fact, it might just make them worse.

Emotional eating tends to leave people feeling "GAMBS" (an acronym for Guilty, Angry, Miserable, Bloated and Sick);- guilty, angry with themselves, miserable, bloated and even a bit sick. It's not a pleasant feeling. If you eat unhealthy food when you feel depressed, you could even get into a vicious cycle where the more you eat, the more depressed you feel, and the more you want to eat.

I can help you to break free, and I want to share a beneficial Cognitive Behavioural Therapy technique explicitly developed for emotional eaters. You can remember it with the acronym **STOP.** Let me walk you through it.

> *"Insanity is doing the same thing again and again, expecting different results".*
> - Einstein.

STOP

Imagine that it's 5.30pm. You have just had a wonderful dinner, perhaps some gorgeous, stir-fried tofu or a delicious salmon steak with hollandaise sauce and a scattering of capers. You are comfortably full, and it was all delicious and healthy. Everything is as it should be.

Then, half an hour later, you find yourself thinking about dessert. You know your spouse has left a slice of cheesecake in the fridge, and it's calling your name. You can't concentrate on what you're doing. All you can think about is that cheesecake. This is where you need to question, are you hungry? Could you be bored? Are you lonely, sad, or craving sugar? Perhaps you're feeling rebellious! Before you head to the kitchen and inhale that dessert:

S - Stop

Stop what you are doing. Take a breath, put down the packet or step away from the fridge. Give yourself room.

T - Take a glass of water and take a pause.

Humans often can't tell the difference between hunger and thirst, so you might find that if you drink a glass of water, you suddenly realise you aren't hungry. This is because hunger creeps up on us slowly, about every four hours. So anything that appears suddenly or less than four hours after a meal is a craving or thirst. Drinking a glass of water also gives you a little more mental space. Also, take a pause. Am I hungry or thirsty? When did I last eat? Am I just bored or sad rather than hungry? What am I feeling?

O - Observe your emotions.

There is a straightforward way to assess whether you are genuinely hungry. First, think of a food you don't like but would eat if you had to. Perhaps jellied eel, offal or even Brussels sprouts. Then ask yourself, would I eat that right now? If the answer is no, you are not truly hungry and know that you have clicked into emotional eating.

Having established that, ask yourself (without any judgement) what emotion you are feeling. It might be immediately apparent, or you might need to take a few moments to let it wash over you until you can identify it. When you are unaware of your emotions, they can control you, but as soon as you identify them, you take away their power. Then, you are back in the driving seat.

P - Plan

Have a plan ready to put into action. For example, you could make a cup of herbal tea to keep your mouth and hands busy or take the dog for a walk to get away from the kitchen. You might combat stress with a hot bubble bath or by turning on the computer and doing some work. Perhaps you phone a friend when you feel lonely or get out a craft or a good book when you feel bored. You could celebrate an achievement with a family dance party or commemorative selfie instead of cake. Whatever plan you want to use, think of a few options in advance so that they are ready and waiting to be put into action when you need them.

STOP is an excellent place to start identifying emotional eating and tackling it. It could take as little as three days to see a shift in your habits and thought processes. But, of course, the problems run deeper for some people and can take them to a much darker place. I use many different tools to help my clients through all sorts of challenges, but I will share just one more with you now. But, of course, there's another acronym to go with it!

RAIN

It would help if you went through this process more than once. A lot of people need to do it five or six times, and some many more than that. You can use RAIN when you know you have a potential challenge, like a party where you'll be tempted to eat or drink more than you want to or to investigate your everyday habits. It can be quite a dark experience, especially if you have trauma to address. Still, reaching the happier and healthier version of yourself is worth it. Once you bring these things out into the open, they don't own you anymore. This is the way to break free.

This is an exercise for your iPhone. Make a new notes section entitled RAIN. Or, for your journal, if you don't have one, grab a sheet of paper to use instead. The space at the end of the chapter might need to be more significant. I want you to write everything you need to, so you might prefer to use a separate sheet of paper and summarise here if you wish. That's entirely up to you.

Start to write following these prompts:

R – Recognise

Let's say it's 7pm, and you've eaten healthily all day. Suddenly you have that craving you might have had for many years, which means you feel you need to have chocolate, crisps or alcohol, for example. As has been your pattern for many years, you have some.

When you eat a chocolate bar, you enjoy it for 2 minutes. For those 2 minutes, it does give you pleasure, and it's OK to acknowledge that. The question is, what happens next? The dopamine rush dies away, and you crave more sugar. Perhaps you eat more. So, you eat more chocolate, more crisps or have another glass of wine. But that fix of pleasure is very short. How long do you feel good? 5 minutes, 10 minutes max? Then as I've said before, for the next few hours, we often feel "GAMBS" - guilty, angry, miserable, bloated and a bit sick. So, you have exchanged 2 minutes of pleasure for 2 hours of feeling sad.

Even the next day, you wake up feeling bloated and regretting your sugary, salty or alcoholic binge. But is that the end of it? Not really! For two weeks, you hate the person you see in the mirror, don't like how your clothes fit and aren't the person you want to be. Each of those chocolate, salty, alcohol binges set off your addiction, and now you can't stop. The cycle continues. Two weeks of misery for two minutes of pleasure.

That's not all. How long have you been overweight? Weight creeps on slowly. It didn't happen overnight. Two years? Two decades?

Two minutes of pleasure for decades of misery. That doesn't sound like a treat. It sounds like hell.

Imagine that you had a best friend who said, "come on, don't be boring, have some Pringles every night! Try the cake I baked. Join me for cheese and crackers." Someone who never stopped pressuring you to eat sugary junk. It's time to realise that this is not your best friend. This is your worst enemy. They have caused years of misery and self-loathing. It's time to break free of that relationship.

Recognise your problem, and then dig deeper to see where it came from. For example, you realise that when you have a hard day at work, you always stop at the shop next to your office to buy a chocolate bar. Do you deserve a treat for a stressful day? but Is chocolate a treat?

Ask yourself, does the food help you? Does it make you feel happy, loved, or whatever you're looking for?

A – Allow

This process can bring up some deep and possibly painful emotions. Allow them to wash over you. Feel whatever you need to feel. Let the realisation sink in. Food is not the answer in this situation. It doesn't resolve more profound issues, and it doesn't make you happy.

This is all not your fault – almost all our eating relationships come from our parents, upbringing, and life experiences.

Now allow yourself to explore a little further. Why do you believe that chocolate is a treat? Why do you associate a chocolate bar with Friday night? You may have to dig deep to get to the bottom of this, and it can take you to quite a dark place, so be kind to yourself and give yourself the time you need.

Your reasons might be simple, perhaps your mother allowed one treat a week, and it was always on a Friday. Or they could be linked to significant trauma and complex emotions. For example, perhaps you were bullied as a teenager and chocolate on the way home was one thing you could control. It could have been a "special treat" that your father gave you when you visited him after a messy divorce. Maybe a good friend used to buy that brand of chocolate, and even though you've lost touch, it makes you feel closer to him.

Perhaps in your mind, alcohol equals happiness? When you were growing up, your parents drank alcohol every night and on holidays, so you associate the two in your mind. But when you have alcohol at home every night, does it bring back those happy memories? Does it get back your parent's love, make you feel as you did as a child growing up with your family or after you've had the alcohol, do you feel even more alone and sad? Allow the reality of your associations to wash over you.

Whatever you discover, let it wash over you without judgement. Once you pull these emotions out into the light, they will no longer have power over you, but allow yourself to experience them for now. This is the old you. As the emotions settle, it's time to say goodbye and welcome a new beginning.

But this is different from your story now. This is your parents' story. You can change this story moving forward. Your life is now your story, not that past life. There is always time to change. Do you want to set your children a better example than the one our parents showed you? Do you want to bring your children up with your eating or drinking addictions, or do you like to correct your story, so they benefit, too, moving forward?

I - Investigate

So now it's time to investigate. To dig deep. Think about the new you. What could you do instead? Could you treat yourself to a magazine instead of food? Track down that old friend? Go for a walk, enjoy a hobby or watch a movie. Think of things that might distract you from food or help you deal with the emotion, and ask yourself what it would take to make you genuinely happy. Do you have any hobbies? My clients who don't have any hobbies or 'me time' are often the ones who have turned to food. They've allowed food or drink to be their pleasure – they derive pleasure from substances rather than finding genuine happiness within themselves.

Think about the person you want to be and the example you want to set for your children (if you have any). For example, do you want to be remembered as someone who was only happy with cake in one hand and a glass of wine in the other? Or do you want to be remembered for genuinely enjoying life and making the most of it?

N - Nurture

This part is beautiful because this is your chance to nurture the new you. You have got rid of the anxiety and the stressful coping mechanisms that didn't serve you. Now you can nurture the new you, who feels happy and spends time with friends and family, being productive or doing things they enjoy instead of turning to food for emotional support. Imagine yourself as that person. Feel what it will be like. See yourself turning away from the chocolate aisle and experience how great it will feel.

Your 'new' best friend says, " Come on, let's watch a movie, play with the kids, phone a friend, and do a jigsaw puzzle. Your new best friend comments that you are fun to be around in the evening. Not that person you used to be who relied on substances (alcohol and chocolate) to make you happy. Your kids now say what a fun parent you are, how you are not the sad parent in the corner relying on substances to provide you happiness. Instead, you have real happiness within.

You may need to go through this process multiple times so take your time. You can return to it whenever you notice a recurring pattern in your behaviour. We all have subconscious motivations, and we can all do RAIN when we want to change our behaviours. I've done it myself, and it is powerful.

If you use STOP in the moment when a craving hits and RAIN to get a big-picture view, then you will have a great toolkit at your disposal to create lasting change. You are powerful, stronger than you realise. You can beat sugar addiction and change your emotional eating habits. Without a shadow of a doubt, those old patterns will soon be behind you, and you will marvel at the way the new you, you imagined is becoming a reality.

I can't wait to see it!

Mindful Eating

You know that there are no rules in RECLAIM your life, but if I had to make one, it would be this: eat at a table. Food is a daytime need, medicine and fuel, but it is also a pleasure. So give it the respect it deserves, enjoy it and fully appreciate it.

If you gave me a box of chocolates while chatting together, I might eat one or two. Give me the same box while watching TV, and I'll eat the whole thing! Most of us are the same. We don't even realise how much we've eaten until we discover the empty box. Not only that, but you also don't really enjoy it either. Really, what's the point of eating if you don't taste the food or even remember eating it? TV eating is mindless eating and is very much linked to obesity.

The same applies to eating standing up. You might nibble on some cheese while you cook or finish the children's leftovers before you do the dishes. Perhaps even sneak into the kitchen for a late evening fridge raid, almost as a kind of me-time. Often my clients need to remember to do these things. They claim they ate nothing other than meals and fruit, and it's only with a bit of digging that they recall the cheese, half a tuna sandwich and a slice of cake.

Eating can be like having a bath. When you're dirty or want to relax, you have a bath. It's a need, and it's also a pleasure. Make it as enjoyable as possible by lighting candles and using special bath salts. Perhaps you linger over your bath for a while. Then it's done, and you get on with your day. You don't try to have a bath and do something else simultaneously. When you need a bath, you have one, you enjoy it, and then you get on with your life.

Eating is the same. You have a physical need to eat, and you can truly experience it, appreciate it and make it a privilege and a pleasure. Plan delicious meals and sit at the table so you can focus as you eat. But you only do it once. After that, you aren't hungry, so you don't need to eat again until your next meal or snack. Instead, you can get on with life!

Positivity and Purpose

What is your purpose in life?

Most of us have several primary purposes:

1. We aim to be financially independent or help our families to be self-reliant.
2. We aim to care for loved ones like children, older relatives, spouses, friends or pets.
3. If we are lucky, we have meaningful work. We know that we make a difference in the wider world, either in a paid or voluntary capacity.

4. Our primary purpose must always be health independence or none of the other 3 will be possible anyway!

All these things give our lives meaning and are the primary substance of our days. To achieve any of them, we need health independence. Just as you don't want to rely on anyone else to support your family financially, you don't want to rely on others to care for your health. So how can you be there for your children (even grown-up children), care for ageing parents, or do your best work if your health fails? Every time you eat a packet of crisps or snacks on a chocolate bar, you are not fulfilling your purpose. But every time you fill up on yoghurt, snack on fruit and binge on delicious healthy foods, you are taking a step towards health independence and being the best you can be.

Please do a little exercise for me. It only takes ten seconds or so! When you wake up every morning, list ten things you are grateful for. It could be anything. There's no need to overthink it. Perhaps you are thankful to be alive and have legs to walk. You could be grateful that your children are safe, that you have a roof over your head or that the fridge is full of healthy food. You could be thankful that the hamster is alive! Just get into the habit of listing ten things each morning, and you will start the day in a beautiful, positive mindset.

Then all you must do is fulfil your purpose. Keep your body healthy to serve you as you do the things you were put on earth to do. That's what makes this program so straight forward. Bingeing on alcohol and crisps is deliberately going against our purpose. We know that. Whereas eating non-processed, non-packaged, non man-made food all day fulfils our purpose. It is as simple as that. So all we've got to say at the end of each day is - did I fulfill my purpose today? That's all we have to do.

> *"I envy the people who stop eating when they're stressed. I'm an emotional eater. I eat my feelings, and unfortunately, they aren't fat-free. They taste a lot like Ben and Jerry's."*
> - Kristen Granata

Dopamine

You know that once you eat sugars, dopamine is released in your brain, which is a feel-good drug stronger than our willpower. As everyone always says, if addiction was just about willpower, there wouldn't be any addicts! So, the best way to avoid cravings is to avoid sugars. It is that simple. Also, the wonderful thing about sugar addiction is that it only takes 3 days for the habit to leave us. Once the sugar is not in our bodies, we don't crave it anymore. I can not tell you how often my clients have started with me on 6 cans of coke or 8 cups of tea a day with sugar. When they come off "the drugs' they say every single time – wow, you were so right; I craved for two days, and by the third day, I didn't want them anymore. The simplest solution, is to say no. Do your STOP and your RAIN, and remember that starting on the chocolates is just going to lead you in the wrong direction, the wrong direction that everybody goes down, not just you. Don't worry. All drugs are designed to make us want more. That is the whole way they are intended.

Put them in the bin.

So next Christmas, Easter or Birthday when you receive that so generous gift (not) of chocolates, you have some choices. Open them, eat them, become addicted again, crave them, want more, keep eating them, finish them, want more, move on to something else sweet… that's one option. Another option is to say thank you very graciously and put them in your fabulous gift cupboard. The first chance you get, make a quick trip to the food bank or charity centre near you and give them away. Or replace the addiction to sugars with the habit of control; take the chocolates, open the bin, shut the bin and feel that power. I promise me that is a wonderful feeling. Pat yourself on the back. I've got this! I'm not an addict anymore. I don't need these. Sugar doesn't control me. Put them in the bin. Put them in the bin. Put them in the bin!

Yasmin, David and Sophie

Yasmin

When she used STOP, Yasmin realised that she often eats when jealous of others or dissatisfied with her life. So the foods she reaches for are the "healthy" treats recommended by lifestyle bloggers and influencers.

Yasmin then used RAIN to try to work out why that was. She realised that when she was bullied as a teenager and started to imitate the "in crowd", thinking that if she looked and behaved like them, the bullies would leave her alone. So she hid her true self behind a mask, tried to blend in, and never quite felt like she belonged in that circle. So she's doing the same thing now, trying to look and behave like the people seen on social media. She hopes to attain their lifestyle and be considered "good enough."

When she pictures a new her, Yasmin imagines doing the things she wants to do. Eating the foods she enjoys and knows to be healthy, wearing clothes she likes and planning the holidays she wants to take - even if they aren't trendy! Feeling confident to be herself and knowing that she is enough just as she is. She is excited to make this new vision a reality!

David

David is the youngest of four brothers and has always wanted to be more significant. His parents could get him to do anything by asking for "a big boy" to help them! Always aiming to catch up with his older brothers, "little Dave" would clear every plate in the hope that it would make him grow big and strong. But, of course, he stopped growing upward long ago and has been growing in a different direction ever since.

David no longer wants to be bigger but wants to be strong, so he has decided to harness that desire. He has come up with a few strategies that he can use as the P in STOP, from simply reminding himself that a packet of crisps won't make him stronger to spending 10 minutes doing some resistance exercises or going for a walk.

Sophie

Sophie didn't even know where to start with RAIN. She sat and stared at the blank paper, feeling lost. She has always been bigger. It's a part of who she is, inextricably entwined with her sense of herself. So how can she pinpoint one trigger or cause for something that big?

Sophie has a lot of threads to untangle, which will not be done in the afternoon.

Instead of trying to work through it all, Sophie has decided to commit to using STOP consistently for 4 days. First, she will note which emotions she identifies as eating triggers (using the notes app on her phone). That will give her a starting point for using RAIN to determine which thread to unpick first. Sophie has also decided when she will do that work, picked a date 5 days from now and written it on the calendar. No excuses!

Over to You

Solutions Bar Test

What are my reactions to the idea of a solution bar? Do they give any clues about my relationship with food?

STOP

These are the plans I will use when I need to stop myself from eating (e.g., a walk, a bath, or phoning a friend):

Having used STOP over a few days, what emotions have I identified as problematic?

RAIN

I have realised this is a problem for me:

Thinking back, it all started when…

The new strategies I can use are:

This is the new me that I want to nurture:

It's time to get out your phone or journal or some blank sheets of paper and start investigating!

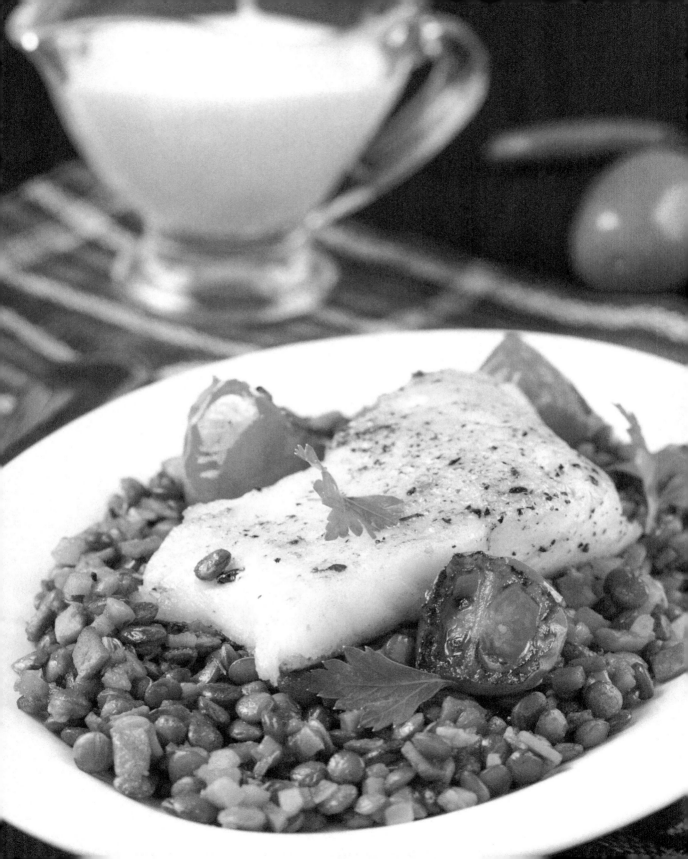

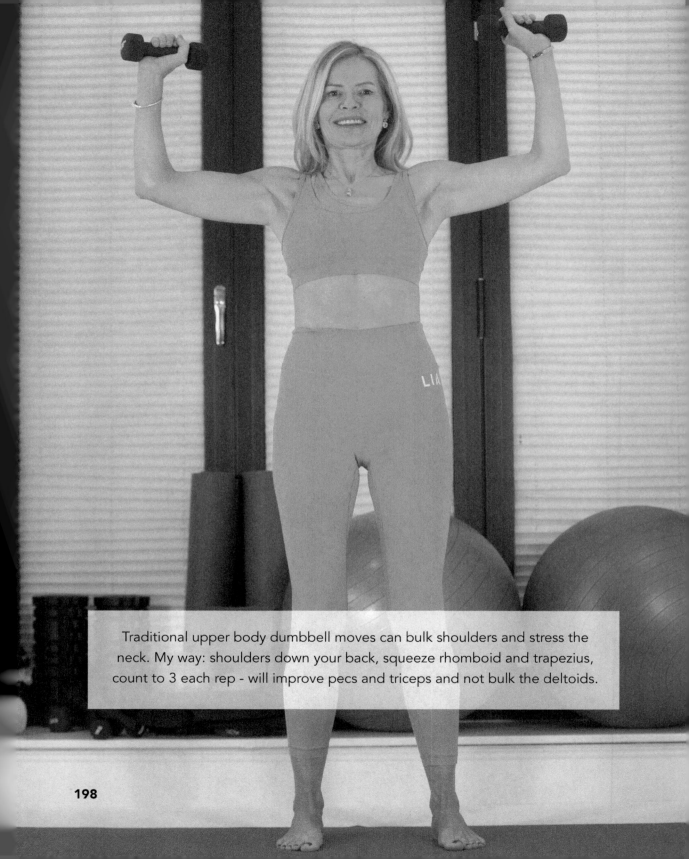

Traditional upper body dumbbell moves can bulk shoulders and stress the neck. My way: shoulders down your back, squeeze rhomboid and trapezius, count to 3 each rep - will improve pecs and triceps and not bulk the deltoids.

M – Movement for Health

"We don't stop playing because we grow old: we grow old because we stop playing." - George Bernard Shaw

The last step in the RECLAIM Your Life in 7 simple steps program is M for Movement. Movement is very important in the weight loss journey. If a nutrition program or ideology doesn't include relevant movement advice, then it should not be considered. We can't achieve a long-term, sustainable, healthy lifestyle without factoring in how much we do and should move each day. This is another reason why so many diet programs don't work. Everybody has a unique metabolism based on their body composition and success can only be truly achieved by understanding all your individual dynamics. That's why your smart scale is so crucial. We need to create the best body composition for the best metabolism eat more and still achieve our body goals!

I like to use the word 'movement' rather than 'exercise' because the whole concept of fitness is terrifying for some people. I want to put your mind at rest here that we don't need to do that much movement to see great results. We certainly don't need to go to the gym or do hours of lactic acid-inducing online HIIT classes!

You'll remember that the body you have now created through three things:

1. 5% is genetics; even that doesn't need to be a life sentence. Although you can't change your height (without taking some unnaturally extreme measures), you can change your body shape, including the size of your thighs, should you want to.
2. 15% of your body comes from what exercise you do.
3. 80% comes from what you eat and drinks.

When you first start your weight loss journey, you will find that the weight falls off when you get your food right. Eat the right foods at the correct times, and the fat will melt away.

However, you might reach a plateau if you don't include much movement in your average week. Many clients want to join my program because they've realised you've gone as far as you can on your own. You've achieved some significant weight loss. Still, you need expert help, particularly in what movement you need to make to get to the next stage in your journey. For example, suppose you aren't moving or you are doing the wrong exercise for your body type or composition. In that case, you will need help to achieve the final stage.

At that point, movement becomes more important. By moving, you can speed up the process of your subcutaneous and visceral fat going down, skeletal muscle going up, and muscle mass going either up or down, whichever you prefer. As a result, movement allows you to achieve whatever shape you want, whether lean and slim or muscular. It's entirely your choice.

Any weight loss or healthy lifestyle program that does not include movement advice like mine will not give you permanent results.

"Ageing is not lost youth but a new stage of opportunity and strength." - Betty Friedan

Visceral Fat

I want to talk about visceral fat first because that is a dangerous type of fat. The fat inside your body is wrapped around your organs and causes many health problems. When you step on your smart scale, you get a reading of 14, 16 or even 30. Ideally, you want to get it down to 6 or below. For someone healthy, that might be as low as 1 or 2. I'm 56 years old, and my visceral fat is 2. You want to focus on this, especially if the number is very high because visceral fat is a killer and reducing it could save your life.

Visceral fat is the main factor in your metabolic age. If you look at your smart scale again, you'll see your metabolic age, the age you have given yourself through your lifestyle choices. If your visceral fat is high, your metabolic age will be much higher than your actual age, perhaps 10 years higher. As your visceral fat melts away, the number will come down, and you might even end up with a metabolic age 5 years younger than you are! Simply losing that fat will add years to your life. Again, although my biometric age is 56, my metabolic age is 45 because of my low visceral fat. It's never too late!

You can achieve this through general movement and low-impact cardio exercise.

> *"If your spine is inflexibly stiff at 30, you are old;*
> *if it is completely flexible at 60, you are young."* -
> Joseph Pilates

Metabolic Age Reversal

My next book will be on my other main 121 program – metabolic age reversal.

Standing v Sitting

The easiest way to add movement to your life is not by going to the gym or doing workouts. It's simply a matter of standing. Can you believe that standing can burn 100 calories per hour?! More people have started working from home in recent years, which is terrific. The problem is that when we used to go to work, we tended to move a lot. You might be walking or standing during your commute, walking through the office, going to the dry cleaners, or even getting a coffee or going to the loo involves walking much further than you do at home. These days many people commute all of 10 feet and then sit on their bottoms all day - no wonder we are gaining weight!

Before the lockdown, the average person did approximately 12,000 steps per day, travelling to work and then moving around the office and meeting areas.

During and after the lockdown, that has reduced to an average of 4,000 steps per day as people work from home. As science states that 3500 calories are equal to 1 lb of fat (on or off), the average person during and since lockdown could have put on as much as 1kg of fat per week (7000 calories). Over all these years, that certainly can add up.

The good news is that you can counteract this without walking laps of the living room. Just standing up makes a huge difference. If you stand for ten hours per day, you can burn 1000 calories and lose 1kg every week simply by standing up! It's incredible the difference it makes. Standing is so important that employers are now under significant pressure to provide standing desks, which raise everything so that employees can work without sitting.

As this is all about health, remember that standing can transform your life in many other ways. For example, standing gives you endorphins which sitting doesn't. Have you ever given a presentation sitting? I don't think so. When you stand, you are alive, and you breathe, and endorphins rush in. When you sit- nothing.

Remember that your head can weigh up to 10 lbs. When you are sitting, your head naturally lolls forwards, pulling on your neck, leading potentially to neck or shoulder aches or even a dowager's hump. However, when you stand, you can put your brain back on top of your spine where it should be with your newly improved standing posture.

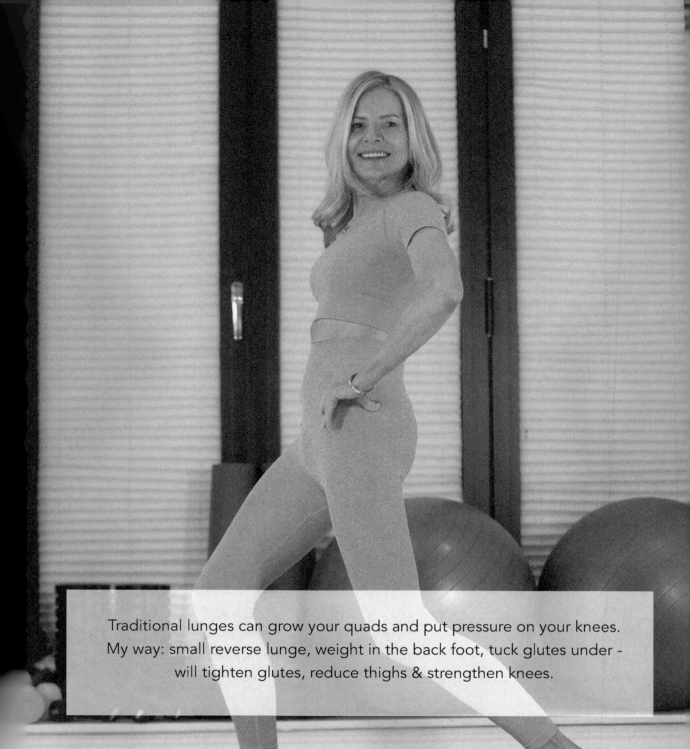

Traditional lunges can grow your quads and put pressure on your knees. My way: small reverse lunge, weight in the back foot, tuck glutes under - will tighten glutes, reduce thighs & strengthen knees.

'A man is as young as his spinal column.'
Joseph Pilates

Additionally, your rhomboids and trapezius muscles in your back assist in holding your pecs (chest) up and firm. When you sit, your pecs can reach your knees! When you stand, you can easily pull your shoulders down your back, naturally improving the lift of your pecs.

You use many of your 650 muscles when you stand, particularly if you pay attention to your posture. Stand tall, with shoulders down, and you will feel your abs and glutes. If you stand as much as possible and sit as little as possible, you have almost done all your daily movement! By standing for 5 hours in the morning, you can have already burned 500 calories. Of course, you'd have to run 5 miles to achieve that. I know which I'd rather do! Remember that the human is a monkey, designed to move, stretch, and climb. We were not made to sit on chairs.

When you sit all day, your muscles are relaxed, your glutes spread, and you might have "lazy glute syndrome". The fat from your bottom might spread out into your thighs. When you stand, can you engage your glutes (bottom)? There is also a risk to your back health if you sit all day, as this is unnatural for the spine. Animals don't sit all day. You have your pelvic floor and spine as bones supporting you. The rest of us is held up by those 650 muscles. Use them or lose them, as the saying goes.

When you sit down, your tummy can only hang out, which can mean your abs might not be engaged the whole day. However, when you stand, you can pull up your pelvic floor (men have a larger pelvic floor than women), and you can see an improvement in your abs definition.

I'm not suggesting suddenly, just standing all day. Standing can be exhausting, so you may want to increase gradually. You are using 650 muscles to hold yourself up, so it's hard work! Start with 20 minutes more than usual and build slowly, perhaps by adding another 20 minutes next week.

I could be pretty extreme here. Of course, it's your choice, and you will need to build up to it, but why not aim at weekdays to almost only sit down to eat breakfast, lunch, fruit snacks and dinner, and in the evening. The rest of the time, stand. If you work at a computer, you can easily buy a standing desk, either a replacement for your current desk or one that goes on top of your existing table. You could even use something like a kitchen island or an ironing board. Both are designed to be used while standing, so they should be at the right height. I use an Amazon iPhone stand wherever I am - £8.99 on Amazon to change your life forever!

Panting

If you want to get rid of visceral fat, then the best thing you can do is low-impact cardio. This exercise that gets your heart beating a little faster at 120 bpm. This needs to be done before breakfast. This is not about pushing yourself too hard. Instead, think naturally. Think only of the intensity levels of dancing, skipping or hopping, a slow jog, a brisk walk, a steady state session on the cross trainer or stationary bike. If you like sports, you can see that tennis players, boxers, cyclists not doing resistance hills, and steady-stage runners have fantastic bodies. They exercise at a rate they can sustain for hours at a time. Sustained, less intense exercise will give you leaner thighs and burn visceral fat. Just enough movement to make you pant, not so much that you are gasping for breath. You should still be able to talk.

One of my favourite ways to do this is boxing. Now I don't mean you must buy gloves and a punching bag, head to the gym or sign up for coaching. Instead, you can use some brilliant YouTube videos at home and for free. Some of my favourites are Team Body Project and Fit Sugar, but there are loads of others. Air boxing is excellent because it tones your arms and strengthens your core but doesn't bulk out your thighs. Of course, if you want muscular thighs, you can also do resistance work to build that muscle. Kickboxing or similar martial arts engages the quads. That is another option if you want to grow your thighs, but regular boxercise doesn't'.

To see good results, scientific research tells us to aim to pant for an hour and a half per week, perhaps split into 30 minutes on three mornings each week. That could mean varying The Body Project low-impact videos each morning or something like walking, tennis or gentle cycling on a Peloton. With low-impact visceral fat burning, the lipids only dissolve whilst we're moving, so when you stop, they stop. I recommend at least 20 minutes per session. Remember that the human body is the greatest invention on the planet. Designed to very cleverly work out the slightest exertion and be ready for battle at a moment's notice. If you do the same low-impact cardio daily, like a dog walk or a walk to work, you will very soon see no new results. It would help if you varied your exercise to keep your body spiked and ready for action.

Traditional mountain climbers people tend to rush & push into their back and thighs. My way: pull belly up, weight forward, wrists under shoulders, count to 3 each move - this will improve abs, triceps and pecs, reduce thigh and back pressure.

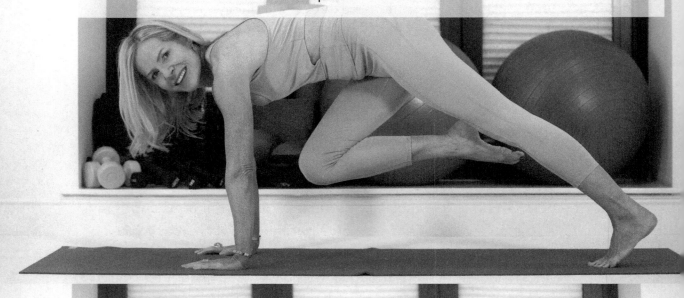

Traditional bicycles don't achieve very much & can hurt the neck! My way: push flexed foot away rather than bring the knee in, keep collar bone open rather than bringing elbow in, push belly button through the floor, count to 3 each rep, keep the chin in chest - this gives outstanding results without growing thighs or stressing neck.

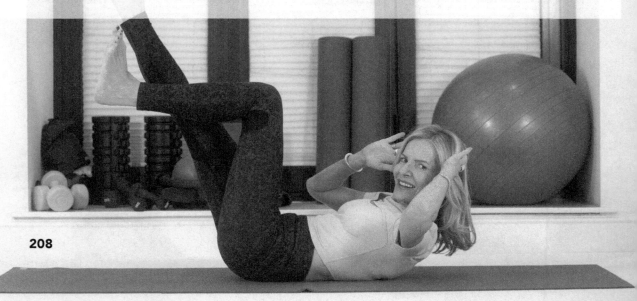

Why mornings? Many suggest exercising in the evenings, but there's a good reason not to do that. When you exercise before breakfast, you have no cortisol in your system. Your body has no other energy source, so it must use your fat stores as fuel. The exercise is quite literally melting away fat. When you exercise in the evening, that doesn't happen. You have eaten, so your body uses sugars as fuel instead of burning fat, which is not the aim! That's great for lactic acid, but we aim to burn fat here. Remember also that HIIT can take your heart up to 190bmp, which is lactic acid burning. Great for fitness, but we are aiming for fat-burning here. We want to work one lower level with the heart at 120 bmp. Another plus is most of my clients are busy working people who don't have the time or motivation to exercise in the evening. Doing it in the morning gets it out of the way!

De-age through exercise

You have 37 trillion cells in your body, and all contain mitochondria apart from the red blood cells. These are the power source of your cells, where the chemical reaction takes place to turn the energy from your food into energy your cells can use. If you imagine each of your cells as a car, you can think of the mitochondria as the engine.

The latest research suggests that you get a new mitochondrion when you exercise in the morning. That's like having a new engine in your car, not just a service or a tune-up but a whole new engine. You become a brand-new Tesla every morning!

It makes sense when you think about it. No animal sits around eating the moment they wake up. Instead, they go out to look for food, wander around grazing, chase down their prey or run away from predators. Humans are only animals, after all, we have done the same thing for thousands of years. Our bodies are designed for this - a bit of panting before breakfast. It makes you feel better, physically and mentally.

So, what happens if you don't exercise one morning? Well, what happens if you never take your car to the garage? Eventually, you have a grotty old engine, spluttering and spewing dirty oil and fumes. This is what happens with your mitochondria. They start pouring free radicals into your body. This causes metabolic ageing, which is why visceral fat and metabolic age are closely linked. So, suppose you exercise in the morning. In that case, you melt away visceral fat and get shiny new mitochondria - your metabolic age could drop by 10 years or more!

It would help if you exercised daily to keep renewing your mitochondria, feeling great, and getting that healthy buzz. The scientific guideline says 3 mornings a week is enough. Still, my clients who work out most mornings have significantly quicker and better results. Just 20 minutes is enough. You could walk to work, or get on the train, tube or bus one stop later or off one stop earlier. Build it into your routine if you can. On three mornings a week, you should concentrate on cardio - anything to make you pant. On the other mornings, focus on resistance exercise (more on that soon), but you can also pant while doing push-ups!

Posture and Slimmer Thighs

Some people, especially men, love having bulky and muscular thighs. But many clients come to me with bigger thighs than they would like, very often caused by posture. If this is a problem for you, don't worry. I have helped a vast number of people to achieve the slender thighs they wanted, and I can do the same for you.

Imagine a person sitting at a desk. Their head is leaning forward, shoulders rounded, and tummy and glutes are hanging out. In that position, they are going to have all sorts of problems. Your head weighs approximately 5kg pulling on your back, causing lots of back pain. When our sitting desk worker stands up, their head is still forwards, still pulling on their back, and it also affects the quads - the muscles at the front of the thighs.

You can quickly test this by standing up. First, stand with your head slightly forward, so your weight is on your toes. Can you feel your quads engaging to hold you up? I call this "quad grabbing", which will bulk up your thighs. Now, stand up straight with your head above your spine. Lift your big toes a little. Did you notice your balance change as your weight shifted backwards? Can you feel that your quads have relaxed? Can you feel your abs now engaging? Can you feel your glutes pulling up and tightening? By putting your weight slightly further back into your heels you've now engaged your glutes and your core. Do this all day, everyday and you will begin to see a noticeable difference as your abs and glutes tighten, lift, and your quads reduce.

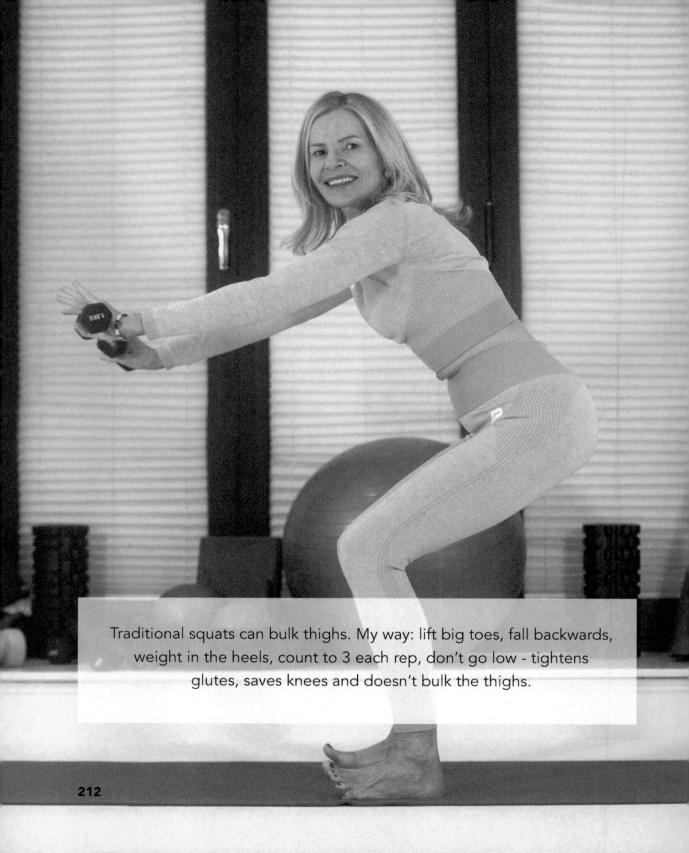

Traditional squats can bulk thighs. My way: lift big toes, fall backwards, weight in the heels, count to 3 each rep, don't go low - tightens glutes, saves knees and doesn't bulk the thighs.

Whenever you stand, stand up straight. Head over the spine, shoulders down, pelvic floor pulled up and even lift your toes a little. Imagine being a ballet dancer or pretending to be a catwalk model. You could even picture yourself as a supremely confident CEO, owning the room as they stride across the office. Good posture is enough to slim down your thighs, but only if you do it consistently. If you struggle, try a posture corrector. They look like a backpack without a bag and are widely available; I recommend one on my website on the recommended products page. Wear one for half an hour daily, and you'll be set up for good posture.

Subcutaneous Fat

The other type of fat, which you will see on your smart scale, is subcutaneous fat. This is the fat that you can see, the one that sits under the skin on your arms, legs and tummy. Subcutaneous fat is less dangerous than visceral fat since it's not wrapped directly around your organs. However, nevertheless, it still has a significant effect on your health. You may want to lose this fat to change your figure. It is mainly caused by SALE: Sugar, Alcohol and Late Eating.

Other than eating the right foods at the correct times, the best way to get rid of subcutaneous fat is through resistance exercise or strength/toning, whatever you prefer. The fat on your body is metabolically inactive -burns no calories, so if this is a high ratio of your body, you will gain weight even if you don't eat very much. If you are lean, with good skeletal muscle and lean tissue but very little fat, then every time you move, you are burning fat. Muscle is metabolically active. Therefore, some people can eat vast quantities of food and never gain weight, while it seems like you only have to look at a cream cake, and you pile on the fat. This is because they have more lean tissue than you, which means they burn fat every moment of the day.

Have you ever wished that you could be one of those people? The friend that everyone finds slightly annoying because they seem to eat whatever they want but stay slim and healthy? The secret is to lose subcutaneous fat and build your skeletal muscles through resistance exercise. As I write this, my son has 10% subcutaneous fat and 60% skeletal muscle. That's 60% of his body burning fat all day long. He can eat pretty much anything he likes!

As you age, it is natural to have some muscle wastage. From around 30 onwards, you can expect to lose 1lb of muscle and gain 1.5lb of fat a year, which starts to show by the time you turn 40. This is natural, but the problem is that as you lose muscle your metabolism shifts. With less muscle, you don't burn fat as you once did, and you gain more and more weight as the years go by, even if you eat the way you did when you were younger. Taking action to build more muscle can reverse that process and turn your body back into a fat-burning machine. Think about it: from 35 - 55 years old, you have lost roughly 20 lbs of muscle and put on 30 lbs of fat. The weight is not the issue, as I always say. The point is that it changes your whole metabolic rate.

It doesn't take hours in the gym to make this change. You have already set aside three mornings a week for panting (burning visceral fat), and you know that you must work out for 30 minutes for that to be most effective. Resistance exercise is quite the opposite! While cardio stops working the moment you stop moving because the lipids stop dissolving the minute you stop moving; resistance exercise burns fat for 72 hours after you stop exercising. That makes it so easy to fit resistance exercise into your day. You can do just a few minutes here and there whenever you have time, or use it as an excellent way to end your day. Resistance exercise is for subcutaneous fat, not visceral, so you don't have to do your resistance moves in the morning, unlike low-impact cardio. Ultimately you are aiming for an hour and a half a week in total of resistance exercise, which could be doing resistance often for a few minutes throughout the day or 20 minutes 4 to 5 times a week, to tone your muscles and melt away that subcutaneous fat. There are 112 hours in a waking week. All I'm recommending is that you give 3 hours of those 112 over to exercise. Is that too much to ask?

I love Pilates. I used to be a Pilates teacher, and yoga is wonderful too but neither of them are useful here unless you add resistance bands. For resistance exercise, you must be pushing or pulling against something, working against resistance. It can be your body weight, some dumbbells, an exercise band, a bottle of water, or a tin of beans. Body weight is an excellent option, not just because it's free and always available but also because it's much heavier than a tin of beans. As always, though, it's your choice.

You can find some excellent videos online. Search for resistance exercises or perhaps resistance exercises on the floor. Good moves include sit-ups, triceps dips, plank, mountain climbers, crunches, glute kickbacks and reverse bridge. If you do resistance as a mesomorph, make sure you do high reps, low weights. I would also like to give you a gift. My exercise video "Toned Arms, Flat Tummy" usually sells for £25 on my website, but you have access for free.

Just use the QR code link to your additional resources page and enjoy the workout. These videos demonstrate how to do resistance exercises safely and effectively.

There are also many resistance videos on my Instagram feed (@ theweightlossgurucom). In addition, I do a live session every Monday and Thursday at 8am GMT. Those lives are all recorded and left on my Instagram feed for you to enjoy for posterity. So, join me for lots of exercise inspiration, motivation and accountability! There are also numerous fitness videos available on my YouTube channel (@theweightlossguru1837).

When you watch my videos, you will see that the movements focus on your arms, legs, tummy and bottom. Of course, when you exercise, you burn fat from all over, not just from whichever part you exercise. Having said that, as the fat melts away, it will reveal the lean tissue underneath. If you have been doing these exercises, that lean tissue will be gorgeously toned.

Squats and Lunges

Squats and lunges are great resistance exercises but avoid them now if you are aim for thinner thighs. This is because most people have been shown how to do squats and lunges by fitness professionals who like being muscular (or were trained by men!). The way you have been taught engages your quads and builds bigger thighs. I can show you another method that doesn't engage your quads, but for now, don't do them. Again, watch my social media to see how to do non-thigh growing squats and lunges if this concerns you.

Your Body Type

Analysing your body type gives insight into which exercise is beneficial for you. Nobody ever fits entirely into one category, and you will almost certainly see elements of yourself in more than one. You may be an equal mix of all three, but many people feel they are 90% one and 10% another, or a 75/25 mix. Whatever you find, it's valuable information.

Ectomorph

Ectomorphs are often thinkers, the stereotype of the writer, inventor or professor. They tend to be long and lean and struggle to gain muscle. Ectomorphs need to focus less on cardio and concentrate on resistance exercises to build muscles. You should build up to quite heavy weights to increase that resistance.

Mesomorph

Mesomorphs are competitive and love to win. Picture the jutting chin and determined gaze of a rugby captain. Although, mesomorphs seem to gain muscle just by looking at a gym. Some women may feel more muscular than they want to be. Mesomorphs who want to reduce bulk should focus on cardio for fitness and avoid too much resistance work.

Endomorph

Endomorphs tend to be easy-going and popular. They love to gather with friends and enjoy delicious food and drink. Picture the convivial host delighting guests with a rare wine or special ingredient. Unfortunately, endomorphs also put on weight quickly and store body fat readily. That was useful in times of feast and famine. Still, in modern Western societies, it leads to a high body fat percentage and often a pear shape. Endomorphs need both cardio to burn fat and resistance exercise to have the lean muscle to burn fat.

Perimenopause and menopause weight gain

As you know, I run whole programs on perimenopause and menopause weight gain solutions. From 35 onwards, we lose that lb of muscle that burns calories, and it gets replaced with the 1.5 lbs of fat that doesn't. Between 35 to 55, therefore, the average woman can lose 20 lbs of metabolically active muscle to be replaced by 30 lbs of metabolically inactive fat. So, the average woman will put on 2 stone between 35 and 55. Then from 55 to 75, we can put on another lb of fat per year around our middle, which are our androgens protecting our organs. But as I say, it doesn't need to be that way! I am 56 years old and 55 kg, but who cares. You can eat and be healthy and look great despite all this if you follow my program. Join me in the under 60 kg club. Join me in the visceral fat under 5 club! These are good clubs to join.

"Ageing is not lost youth but a new stage of opportunity and strength." - Betty Friedan

HRT – Hormone Replacement Therapy

We are all entitled to our own opinions. That is the beauty of being in this justice system rather than a dictatorship. From my personal experience, I think HRT is a lifesaver, and it has been to many of my thousands of clients. I have yet to see any adverse effects from this women's life saver and positively

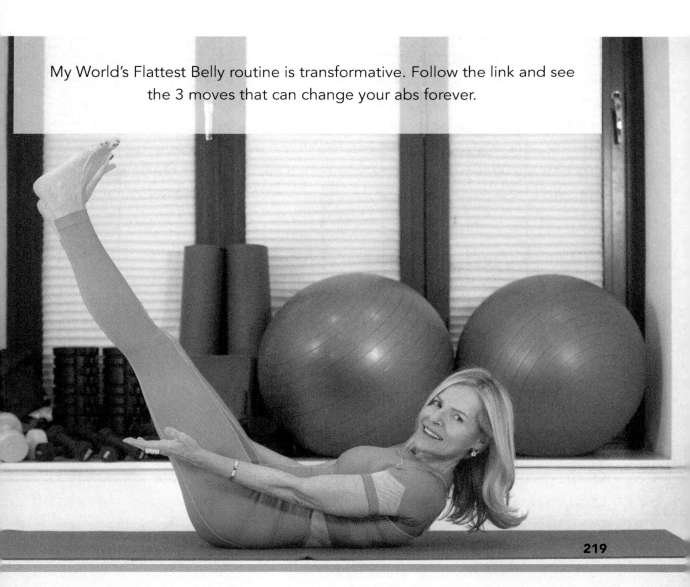

My World's Flattest Belly routine is transformative. Follow the link and see the 3 moves that can change your abs forever.

endorse it. But only because one size does not fit all in today's world. In previous generations, HRT was a once size fits solution. What happens if you've got very high levels of progesterone, and testosterone and yet zero oestrogen? A one size fits all solution would have been a disaster.

When I first went to get tested, aged 53, in the middle of a terrible marriage that I was trying to escape, I was told by a male doctor that I had depression and put straight onto Sertraline, the anti-anxiety medication. Now Sertraline is a wonderful miracle cure for many clients suffering from low anxiety or depression. I recommend it for anyone going through a bad phase in their life and not coping, and I would also recommend staying on it if it helps. If they take your hand off you and offer you another one, why wouldn't you take it? The ridiculous stigma around mental health makes me so angry – particularly after how my father was treated until he tried taking his own life three times. The third time was successful. So I have no complaints about Sertraline at all.

However, in this instance, when I went to that male doctor, feeling a bit down and not sleeping well at the age of 53 was classic menopause symptoms. So I went back and saw a female doctor who immediately agreed. I requested to have my oestrogen, progesterone and testosterone levels tested. Get all three tested every time, as you need to know what it is you're up against.

Low progesterone – low libido, hot flushes, depression, sore breasts, low blood sugar, absence of menstrual cycle.

Oestrogen – dry skin, night sweats, moodiness, irritability, poor concentration, irregular periods, brittle bones,

Testosterone – reduced sex drive, loss of armpit or pubic hair, hot flashes

Look at all these symptoms that can be reversed simply by a merino coil and rubbing some gel onto it once a day! Crazy.

I had zero progesterone and zero oestrogens. My testosterone, if anything, is slightly high. That is why HRT is never one size fits all. So literally half of my personality, half of me, had been taken. Once on the Mirena coil and Oestrogel, I have been tickety-boo ever since. My happiness, positivity, laughter and love of life have returned. I was lucky I never suffered from low libido or sex drive. Still, I did experience some of the other symptoms, such as irritability and night sweats. Since being on HRT, all of these have vanished, and I've got my mojo back on – fully!! So please, the minute you experience any of the above, even when you are just in your 40s – you don't get a reward for being a hero – see a doctor and get yourself sorted!

Menopause and Weight Gain

From a weight loss perspective, these blood tests are also crucial. Oestrogen lubricates your joints, and any deficiency can lead to inflammation within the body. Remember the 3 causes I mentioned that can increase the fullness of your fat cells - insulin inducing foods, stress and inflammation. Suppose you're losing weight more slowly than you expect. In that case, it could be that your oestrogen levels are low; therefore, your body has inflammation = adrenaline = glucose = weight gain. If you have inflammation, you can not lose weight.

So go to the doctor and get your blood tested – if it's worth it to change your life for the better. Your health is your wealth. Don't forget to invest in yourself.

Make sure you get your blood tested if you experience the first sign of perimenopause. Please don't leave it too late.

Yasmin, David and Sophie

Yasmin

Yasmin has always hated her thighs and couldn't understand why her hours in the gym made no difference. Now she realises that she's 70% mesomorph and 30% endomorph. So those big thighs are mostly muscle!

Yasmin has set the alarm to get up early three days a week and do some boxing before she goes to work. She loves that boxing focuses on her arms and core rather than her legs. Yasmin has also stopped doing lunges and squats and will be careful not to bulk up her arms too much.

Yasmin is also going to ask her manager about getting a standing desk.

David

David was the stereotypical weedy little kid who always wanted to be bigger. He thinks he might be 50% ectomorph and 50% endomorph, gaining weight quickly but struggling to build muscle. He has scheduled some time for cardio, but his focus is on resistance and muscle building. David is considering investing in some weights to make the most of his resistance work. Still, he is doing lots of exercises that use body weight instead.

222

Sophie

Sophie thinks she's probably about 90% Ectomorph and 10% Mesmorph. She feels she'll have to "throw everything at it" to get the desired results. Sophie plans to walk to school every day, 10 minutes in each direction. On three days a week, she'll walk a bit further to get 30 minutes of cardio while her little ones are safely strapped into the buggy. If it's pouring rain, Plan B is to head home and follow PIppa's resistance and strength videos on Instagram and also the free videos she's given in this book to ensure she's doing all the exercises the correct way. She'll do this twice per week during weekdays for 30 minutes and then one extra 30 minutes session over each weekend.

"Researchers find exercise often works just as well as drugs for the treatment of heart disease and stroke, and the prevention of diabetes. Exercise is medicine." - Dr. Michael Greger

Over to You

Grab your phone or journal and make plans to get moving this week. You might like to answer these questions:

My body type is:

My particular problem areas (e.g., bulky thighs or low muscle tone) are:

The type of exercise I need to concentrate on is:

This week my cardio plan is as follows:

And I will do this resistance exercise:

Now You're Successfully
On The Plan –

"It's often said that when the fear of staying the same outweighs the fear of change, that is when we change." - Jay Shetty

How to stay on it.

Using the seven simple steps, you now have all the information you need to change your life forever. Then, all you must do is put it into action! But, of course, we all know it's more complex than that, so to help you reclaim your life and make your dream a reality, I have one last acronym for you. So, get out your phone or journal, or turn to the end of this chapter, and start to GROW.

7 Day Challenge

Once you've got all the knowledge, all the food recommendations and timings, all the recipes, all the nutrition knowledge, emotional eating help and exercise advice relevant to your body type, you can start the program. It will work to give you incredible results. At this stage, it is beneficial to set some goals and challenges, both weekly and more long-term, to motivate you to stay on plan and reward yourself each week you successfully make good decisions and the right choices. Here are a few goal-setting strategies and mechanisms to not only keep you on your journey successfully but also so that you can congratulate yourself every day. This will keep you focused until the successful results' momentum carries you through.

For example, a typical 7-day challenge for a new reclaimer is here.

- 4 mornings x 4 ticks 20 minutes panting before breakfast
- 3 evenings x 3 ticks 20 minutes resistance exercise after dinner
- 7 days x 7 ticks conscious of standing more (buy standing desk)
- 7 days x 7 ticks 2.5 litres of water a day
- 5 days x 5 ticks eating dinner before 7pm
- 5 evenings x 5 ticks, no alcohol
- 6 days x 6 ticks, no rubbish snacks
- 7 days x 7 ticks no eating standing or telly eating

GROW

G - Goals

Do you remember in chapter 1 when you committed to your new future? What did you want to achieve? Renew that commitment by choosing three or four goals and writing them down. Some possible plans might be:

- To fit into the clothes that you haven't worn for years
- To hit a specific target weight
- To run a marathon
- To get off medication

- To be pain-free
- To be more confident
- To buy clothes in high street shops

Goals are very individual. There are no right or wrong answers here, so long as you feel excited about the future.

R - Reality

Be honest and describe your current reality. Nobody else ever needs to see this page, but it's essential to know the truth yourself. For example, you might write about your current weight, describe symptoms you want to get rid of or talk about your lack of confidence.

This step might be painful now, but it will be fun to look back and see how everything has changed! In just a few short months, you won't be able to believe that what you write here was ever true.

O - Options

O defines your options for creating change, and that's easy! Just follow the 7 most straightforward steps in the world.

- Real food - fill your fridge with natural, unprocessed foods and enjoy the most delicious meals you have ever eaten. Focus on a healthy balance of proteins, non-sugary carbs and good fats as we've planned.

- Eating times - the key to lasting change. Eat breakfast as late as you can (about 10 or 11) and dinner as early as you can (around 5 or 6)

- Cut out the junk - simply replace the starchy grains with pulses!

- Liquids - water is the source of all life, so drink enough. Enjoy no more than two cups of tea or coffee daily, and try to drink them black or with just a dash of milk. Be careful of milk, smoothies and juices.

- Alcohol - no more than two units, on two nights a week.

- Investigate - explore the emotions behind your actions. For example, discover how to enjoy food without letting it rule your life.

- Movement - burn fat all day by standing rather than sitting, use cardio to lose visceral fat and resistance exercise to tone muscles and melt subcutaneous fat away.

W - the Will and the Way

How strong is your will to make this happen? On a scale of 1 to 10, 1 means that you don't care and 10 means you are determined to be unstoppable. You need this number to be 8 or above. If it's not, then look again at your goals and reality. Do you need to change your plans? Turn back to chapter 1 and peek into the magic mirror once again. Consider your purpose in life and how much better you can fulfil your goal if you are strong and healthy. Use the RAIN technique from chapter 8 to see what is holding you back.

Once your will is strong enough, you can map your way forward. What will you do this week to put everything you have learnt into practice? I don't want you ever to feel pressured or restricted, don't fall into "all or nothing" thinking and feeling that if you can't do everything, you might as well give up. If 30 minutes of exercise feels too much, can you do 5 minutes? Could you eat early on two nights this week or cut out two pasta bowls? Don't worry about doing everything. Just plan one baby step that you can take this week.

It would be helpful to ask someone to be an accountability buddy, whether you check in online once a week or eat lunch with them every day.

It's also helpful to think about when you will look for feedback and decide what to do next. As you have worked through this book, you will have noticed that I often give you several options to choose from or set different challenges, and you might like to try out more than one possibility. A good time to review is once a week when you weigh yourself. Take a minute to reflect on what has gone well and what hasn't. How do you feel? Are the numbers on your smart scale moving the way you want them to? Do you want to take on a new challenge or another baby step in the coming week?

What's Next?

In this book, I have given you a good grounding in creating a lifestyle that will work for you and help you reclaim your healthy, happy life. However, I am aware that every book has its limitations. I don't know you personally, and I can't offer tailored advice or give you accountability.

You can take the information you read here, apply it and reach your goals. If that's you, then congratulations! I would love to celebrate with you, so please share your success story by tagging me on social media or sending me a message.

Some readers, however, will need more support or something more in-depth. That's fine. This is a complex topic, and making a change can be difficult. If that's you, here are some other ways I can help you.

Reclaim Your Life 1-2-1 program

If you enjoyed this book but need some personal help to put it all into action, this option could be perfect for you. This program has similar content to what you have here but with lots more videos and personal support. You will have one-to-one sessions with me weekly and access to my private client-only Facebook group for life.

Metabolic Age Reversal Program

If your focus is on health, you might be interested in this program, which comprehensively covers metabolic age reversal. If your metabolic age exceeds your actual age, I can show you how to reduce it by 10 years more! As a result, reverse the symptoms of many health conditions and reduce the risk of others developing. This program is life-changing and lifesaving!

1-2-1 sessions

Whatever you need help with, you can book a session with me. We will meet via video call, and I can support you. For example, go deeper into your emotional response to food, get my help planning the right exercise program, or discuss how to maintain your new figure. I am available to answer any questions and help you RECLAIM your life. Just get in touch for more information.

As I write this, I have 20 nutrition and 15 exercise videos available for you to buy from my website for just £10. So, whether you want to know more about how female hormones influence weight loss or need a new workout, there's bound to be one to suit you! You can find them all in my shop.

Of course, the services I offer may change over time as I develop new programs and record new videos. However, you will always find up-to-date information on everything currently available on my website theweightlossguru.co, and you can also contact me there.

Yasmin, David and Sophie

Yasmin

Yasmin's GROW

Goals: Lose 5kg, slim down my thighs and gain enough confidence to apply for a new job.

Reality: I weigh 81kg and have a BMI of 29. I struggle to find trousers that fit well. They always feel tight around my thighs. Trying to lose weight has dominated my life, from hours spent at the gym to trying whatever diet the latest influencer recommended. As a result, I don't measure up, and I don't have much confidence.

Options: 7 simple steps!

Way Forwards: This week, I will eat at 11am, 2pm and 4pm each day, enjoying lots of delicious foods. I will move my regular gym sessions to the morning and focus on cardio - no squats or lunges! I am also going to try drinking on Friday night only. I will ask my sister to be my accountability buddy and send her my results when I weigh in each week.

6 months later

What a transformation! Yasmin lost her excess fat within a few weeks. It took a little longer to slim down her muscular thighs, but she persevered and now has the lean figure she always wanted. More than that, Yasmin has stopped lusting after the lifestyles seen on social media. She no longer feels like a second-rate copy of Instagram influencers. Now she has taken control of her own life.

Yasmin knows that she has the power to create the body she wants, strong, healthy and looking great! She no longer worries about what to eat or how to deal with special occasions. It's all so simple. She continues living healthily, following her new lifestyle without a second thought.

This success has given Yasmin the confidence boost she needed. She bought a fabulous new interview outfit that makes her feel on top of the world. Yasmin is yet to find her dream job, but only because she's being picky. In the past, she would have accepted anything to get out of that cubicle. Now she knows her worth and has even turned down a few roles that wouldn't have made her happy.

Yasmin knows it's worth waiting a little longer, and she does not doubt that her dream job is just around the corner.

Dave

David's GROW

Goals: Lower my blood sugar to non-diabetic levels. Lower my visceral fat to 9. Not get out of breath at work.

Reality: My visceral fat is 16, and my metabolic age is 67 - 10 years older than I am. My blood tests showed that I was pre-diabetic. I got so out of breath at work that a patient joked I would need an oxygen mask.

Options: Follow the steps in Reclaim your life

Way Forward: I'll start with the no-cook meal plan, then try out a few of Pippa's recipes once I've got my confidence with this way of eating. I'm not too fond of the sound of those parasites, so no more beer. Next, I will order some weights for resistance exercises. Finally, I've told my colleagues in the ambulance that I'm on black coffee or water only - they will never let me hear the end of it if they catch me with a toffee latte!

6 months later

When David walked into the GP surgery for a follow-up blood test, his doctor could hardly believe her eyes! The man standing in front of her looked like a picture of good health, nothing like the David she had warned 6 months previously.

It took David 5 months to melt away the fat. He lost 28 kg, but his visceral fat and metabolic age were the numbers he liked to watch drop. His metabolic age went down 14 years - now, his body is younger than he is!

David/s blood tests last week came back normal. He doesn't have to take any regular medications anymore and feels full of energy. He rarely gets breathless at work these days. He has even joined a Saturday morning football club, where he regularly outruns some younger men!

Sophie

Sophie's GROW

Goals: To have a healthy BMI and see it turn green on the smart scale app. To walk into any high street shop and know they will stock my size. No longer be the fattest mother at the school gate. Have more energy.

Reality: I need to lose about 40kg, and my body is over 40% fat. All my clothes must be ordered online from specialist shops, and often they could be better when they arrive. I am always the biggest person in any room and worry about fitting into chairs.

Options: RECLAIM my life!

Way Forward: Start eating with the children at 5pm. Make a point of sitting down to enjoy meals, even if it's just me, and don't eat toast or sandwiches! Imagine I'm in a posh restaurant, no cereal here.

6 months later

Sophie has transformed her life and is well on the way to reaching her goal. In 6 months, she has lost 32 kg, and while her BMI might not be green on the app, it has gone from red to orange, which is a great start. Sophie loves her new lifestyle; it doesn't feel like any of the diets she had tried before. Sophie never feels restricted and knows she will continue to live this way forever. Nothing can stop her from reaching her goal; especially now it's only 8 kg away!

Sophie's children love having a newly energetic mother. So Sophie started looking for ways to include more movement into her day instead of sitting and watching them play. They run around together at the park, have dance parties in the kitchen, and even plant a small vegetable garden. Sophie loves that when someone suggests a trip out, she can say, "let's go", instead of feeling that she would rather be asleep on the sofa.

Sophie's biggest win was the day she saw a nice top for sale in the supermarket. She was delighted to discover that they had her size in stock, and it's now her favourite top. Since then, Sophie has been to a few high street shops and loves being able to try things on before she buys them. So she's saving up for a new wardrobe when she hits her goal!

Over to You

It's time to get out your phone or journal and ponder the following:

How will I make this happen?

- My Goals
- My Reality
- My Options
- My will, on a scale of 1-10
- My Way Forward
- Do I need to ask anyone to keep me accountable? Who? What do I want them to do?
- When will I check in, review my progress and make any tweaks needed?
- Put a reminder on the calendar!

You are now ready to transform your existence. To become the person you want to be, living in a body you love. This is a beautiful journey, and I am both honoured and proud to walk alongside you as you reclaim your life.

I know that you are going to achieve your goals. I guarantee that you will feel better every single day that you follow this plan. But if you ever need extra help, know I am here. Reach out on social media or have a look at my website. I'm here to help.

Pippa Hill

(The Weight Loss Guru)

Free Bonus – Food Planning Inspiration

As I mentioned in chapter 5, I'm always reluctant to give people meal plans. It's easy to see a plan and think you must stick to it when the reality is that success has very little to do with rigidly following someone else's menu and a lot more to do with mindset and a genuine understanding of how to nourish your body for good health.

Many people find it helpful to have some examples of meal plans just so they can see how everything might fit together, for a bit of inspiration or to use if they don't have time to plan. So, as a bonus, I am giving you five different meal plans and 101 recipes, more than enough to get you into the swing of things.

Please don't treat these plans as prescriptions. Instead, change them, swap out meals you don't like and add in your favourites, or mix them up and have a meat-free Monday and no-cook Wednesday. Use the 5 different food plans with the 58 delicious recipes to create your perfect way of eating as you reclaim your body, health, happiness and life.

I have included plans for people who eat everything, vegetarians, vegans, and pescatarians, a no-cook plan and one for those eating a fruit dinner. There should be something for anyone, and the food truly is delicious, even if I say so myself. I can't wait to hear your thoughts and see the fabulous results you get as you RECLAIM your life.

Scan the QR code to download your fantastic free meal plans and recipes:
Your password is TWLGBOOKRYL

Acknowledgements

Writing a book is a huge undertaking, not something anyone can do alone. So, as ever, there are many people I want to thank. Starting with my three children, who consistently put up with my obsessive passion to save the world from obesity!

Thank you to Lorna (@growing_business_and_babies / wordsbylorna.com) for her word skills and poignant insights into how lacking confidence in our body can profoundly affect many. Thank you to Marina (@nutriprep_kitchenuk / nutriprepuk.co.uk) for her beautiful food plans design and for all the support in publishing this book. Thank you to Thalie for being a great assistant. I want to thank Julian Christopher Paul Eden MBBs Bachelor of Science MRCGP for his scientific checks and to Phil (@parklifephotographylondon / philwilsonphoto.co.uk) for his fabulous photos.

Finally, but most importantly, thank you to all my clients for their commitment to improving their lives and unwavering support for this program.

I couldn't have done it without you all.

About the Author

Ranked as one of the top weight loss experts in London, Pippa Hill, The Weight Loss Guru has poured 43,000 hours of evidence-based experience into her new book Reclaim Your Life (in 7 simple steps).

As a Nutritionist, Eating Psychology Coach and Exercise expert, Pippa has developed this proven program using her many years of experience. With it, she helps over 1000 clients permanently achieve the healthy lifestyle they aspire to every year.

Discover more ways to work with Pippa at https://theweightlossguru. co/get-started/

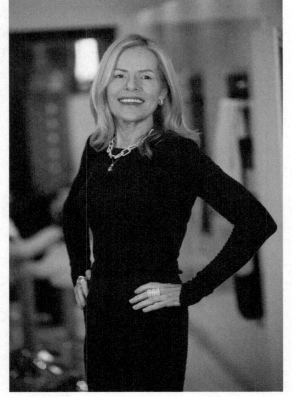

Printed in Great Britain
by Amazon

23694931R00143